The Dizzy Patient

The Balance System and Dizziness

by
Soren Vesterhauge, MD, DMSc,
Copenhagen, Denmark

ISBN-13: 978-1537789989

CONTENTS

1. PREFACE

My background is that of a medical doctor (MD) trained in Otolaryngology (ears, nose and throat - ENT) and Aviation Medicine. I have a broad approach to the ENT-specialty, including experience in almost all kinds of ENT-surgery and student teaching as a senior lecturer. The focus on my involvement in Aviation Medicine has been otolaryngology, and for a short period of six months I served as a chairman of the Civil Aviation Medicine Clinic in Copenhagen.

I have conducted scientific research, particularly in the field of balance function in zero-gravity along with technician Pernille Mikines and our engineer, Arne Månsson. In the 1980th we conducted several series of parabolic flights experiments (weightlessness achieved by a parabola trajectory flight pattern) heavily supported by grants from the Danish Space Foundation, very much facilitated by a donation of a large number of flying hours by the Royal Danish Air Force (RDAF). Some of the research was made in a collaboration with ESA (European Space Agency) or NASA.

My background in the field of *vertigo and disorientation in flight* was supported by demonstrations and discussions with Kent K. Gillingham, MD, PhD and James W. Wolfe, PhD during a number of visits to US Air Force School of Aerospace Medicine, Brooks Air Force Base, San Antonio, USA, and by discussions with my Danish colleague, Thorkil Fussing MD, who was never satisfied with an imprecise conclusion. Teaching vertigo and disorientation in the RDAF for more than 20 years drove me into the depths of the topic.

My insight into some of the puzzles of basic balance physiology is a consequence of meeting and learning from, first of all my American friend, the great balance physiologist Professor Dennis P. O'Leary PhD, and from encounters with a large number of other great people from the international league of balance research from countries such as Sweden, the USA and Great Britain, (to name a few: Professor N.G. Henriksson MD of Lund, Professor Jan Stahle MD of Uppsala, Dr. Alan J Benson PhD of Farnborough and Owen Black MD of Portland, Oregon, who taught me about the posttraumatic perilymphatic fistula).

A deep insight into basic balance physiology is an indispensable base of handling and understanding dizzy patients. For more than 25 years, Pernille Mikines and I had the pleasure of running a dizziness clinic at the University Hospital, *Rigshospitalet*, in Copenhagen and later in a private hospital.

The text in this book may be considered more or less controversial for the following reasons:

5

1. There are no specified scientific references. Reasons: Scientific referencing is a diverse field. There are always a large number of relevant references. Most authors face a choice between quoting those references that fit their purpose and omitting those that do not, or on the other hand choosing from both shelves in order have a balanced and intelligent discussion.

The consequence of my choice is, that the form of the present book is closer to that of an essay than to that of a textbook or scientific survey of the topic – focusing on my own experiences.

2. In the present work, there is a bias towards a description of peripheral (i.e. related to the sensory organs) phenomena. It is my experience that it is relevant.

This book is written for anyone interested in the topic, including those professionally faced with dizzy patients (i.e. medical specialists, nurses and physical therapists), as well as dizzy patients who are searching for more insight into dizziness and vertigo.

Copenhagen, October 2016
Soren Vesterhauge, MD, DMSc

2. INTRODUCTION

When studying *balance physiology*, there is no doubt of the conclusions drawn. The king and the queen of the sensory organs involved are the *vestibular organs* of the inner ear, the *otolith organs* (the *saccule* and the *utricle*), and the *semicircular canals* (three canals in each ear).

Without information about the direction of gravity and information about own motions, balance does not work. This is probably why the most frequent causes of vertigo and dizziness are found in different types of dysfunctions of the vestibular organs of the inner ear.

When talking about *orientation*, i.e. the unconscious registration of surroundings, including people, and objects around us and their motions, the balance system relies on a joint venture with other sensory organs, first of all vision and hearing. Orientation may be considered balance in a much broader sense.

When considering *locomotion*, very important sensory information (proprioception and kinesthesia) from muscles and joints about contraction, motion and the position of head, trunk, and limbs as well as pressure sensations from the soles of our feet all joins the balance venture.

Therefore, any deeper approach to dizziness and balance problems must involve knowledge of the normal sensory physiology and the data processing of that information in the brain. These are the fundamentals and logic of this book.

Once these fundamentals have been covered, the next step in understanding dizziness and vertigo is to study what can go wrong in the sensory organs and the brain that can lead to dizziness and balance disturbances, and how can we cure it.

Last but not least, we must also be aware of the psychological reactions to dizziness and balance problems. This is dealt with in the last chapter of this book.

3. A PRESENTATION OF THE BALANCE SYSTEM

Anatomy and physiology of the balance system are both rather complex. For the human species, in particular, high demands are made to the balance system due to our upright position and bipedal behavior. The system's function is based on collaboration between a number of sensory functions among which the otolith organs and the semicircular canals play a major role. The conductor of the orchestra is real world experiences with successful and less successful balance performance stored in the central nervous system (CNS). Gravitation is the main leading instrument in this symphony, since any shift in position or motion must be harmonized with the gravitational pull.

Insight into balance physiology is a prerequisite of the understanding of dizziness and vertigo.

3.1 The physical basis of the function of the balance system

The balance system is one of our biological responses to being forced to live in the gravitational field of our planet.

3.1.1 Gravitation

Mountains are constantly eroding because rain and rivers, subjected to the influence of gravity, transport material from the mountains towards the valleys.

Oysters must stay on the ocean floor.

Birds must use the force of their wings to stay airborne.

A blade of grass and a tree both have primitive sense organs telling them about the direction of the gravitational pull, so their growth becomes vertical, rather than creeping randomly along the surface.

Humans know what is up and down - we know the rules of the game. If we, standing or moving on our legs, lose control of up and down, we fall. It is part of our life condition. The very few who know what it is like to be weightless for a while and then return to gravity, e.g., the astronauts, describe it as a heavy burden. For the great majority of us, gravity is our destiny and is lived out, far from our daily attention.

From science, we now know more about the true nature of gravitation, which has always been an unsolved riddle, even though it has been known for some time that the effect of gravitation can be compared to an upward acceleration at a rate of 9.8 m/s^2 if there was no gravitational pull. This is strange because gravitation is not motion, but a force directed towards the center of the earth that defines our contact with our earthly foundation. In an elevator accelerating upwards or decelerating downward, we can feel a force added to the gravitational force; on decelerating upwards or accelerating downwards, the gravitational pull is reduced. If you are in doubt, bring your bathroom scale along on your next elevator ride.

A rocket or any other object designed to travel upwards must produce a force higher than that resulting from a 9.8 m/s^2 vertical acceleration.

3.1.2 Navigation

Our survival is not only dependent of our strategies to overcome the effects of gravity it is also dependent on our opportunities to move around on the surface of our planet. Gravitation offers us a relatively firm physical contact to the surface and delivers friction that usually allows us to walk, run and under other conditions to ski, skate or skid, depending on the footwear and the quality of the surface. What we need to be able to navigate, is to make use of aids that can be compared to the navigational instruments used by the shipmaster when navigating his ship:

1. You need a *chart*. In this case, the chart is deposited in a structure of the more primitive part of the brain called the *hippocampus*. Even a feeble old man is able to find the bathroom half-asleep in the middle of the night under poorly lit conditions in his own home. The route is well charted in his *hippocampus*. If he is away from home, the procedure must be carried out a number of times with our gentleman fully awake and with all lights on before the route is well charted in the hippocampus.
2. There is a need of a compass to ensure a precise and steady heading under less clear visual conditions (in aviation termed "instrument flight conditions"). This service is provided by the *semicircular canals,* recording angular movements of the head, more or less easily integrated into position. Almost every normal person is able to walk straight ahead with their eyes closed or blindfolded, thanks to the canals. Under ideal visual condition, the canals further guarantee eye movements compensating for the unavoidable head movements caused by walking or running, and thus ensuring a stable visual direction.
3. The shipmaster must control the torque of the engine or the function of the sails in order to maintain a steady or at least controlled speed of the vessel. In human locomotion, this function is handled by a careful trimming of muscular activity, considering both the pull of gravity and the aim of the motion, carrying the individual from point A to point B. This is really complex brain work starting with a more or less conscious intension to

move the distance and ending with a safe arrival. This is much more complex than the captain's task with the ship's engine order telegraph.

3.2 Sensory organs of the inner ear involved in the balance

The king and the queen of the sensory organs of the balance system are located in the inner ear.

The *otolith organs* report the direction of the gravitational pull and the *semicircular canals* keep track of head motions. The otolith organs are sensitive to the gravitational pull and forces created by linear accelerations. The semicircular canals respond to turning motions of the head. The otolith organs are not uninfluenced by turning motions of the head, since such motions result in linear centripetal and tangential accelerations. It means that the two types of balance organs of the inner ear have overlapping functions.

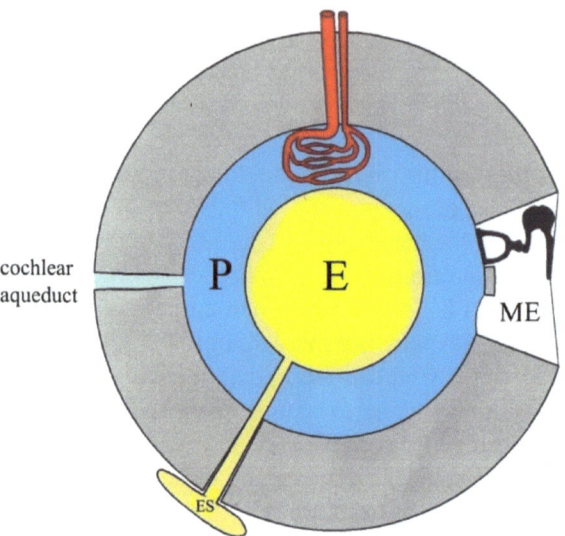

*Figure 3.1. Schematic view of the inner ear. It is surrounded by the hard bone of the skull. There are two fluid filled spaces, the **perilymphatic space** (P) filled with the sodium rich **perilymph** and connected to **the cerebro-spinal fluid** via a tiny canal called the **cochlear aqueduct** (left). The inner space is the **endolymphatic space** (E), containing **endolymph**, rich in potassium. The perilymphatic space is separated from the air-filled middle ear (ME) by the foot plate of the stapes, the surrounding joint of the stapes and below that by an elastic membrane in the round window.*

The sensory organs are well protected within a cavity in the part of the temporal bone called the **petrous bone**. The bone is very hard compared to other bones in the body but, but unlike other bones, it does not grow or change its shape.

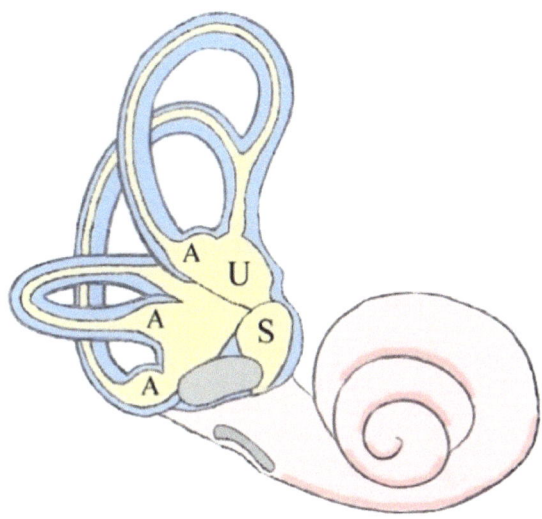

*Figure 3.2. The inner ear. Posteriorly there are three **semicircular canals**, each perpendicular to the two others. These are the **horizontal canal**, the **superior canal**, and the **inferior canal**, respectively. They meet in a cavity called **the vestibulum**. The canals all have a small dilation in one of the ends attached to the vestibulum (A). This is called the **ampulla** and contains the sensory organ of the canal, the **ampular organ** (fig. 3.7). Intimately connected with the canal system there is **the utricule** (U), a small saclike structure containing one of the otolith organs. The other otolith organ, **the saccule** (S) is anatomically more related to the cochlea. All together they are the **vestibular organs.***

It is similar to a set of Chinese boxes filled with a fluid of the same composition as the fluid surrounding brain and the spinal cord (the **Cerebro-Spinal Fluid, CSF**). In the inner ear, the fluid is called the *perilymph*. There is a tiny canal connecting the perilymphatic space with the CSF space. Included in the perilymphatic space there is another space, the *endolymphatic space*, surrounded by a tiny, but very active membrane. The endolymph is characterized by a high concentration of potassium, whereas the perilymph as any other body fluid is rich in sodium. This difference in chemical composition results in an electric potential like the potential difference characteristic of a battery. The membrane houses the sensory cells of the inner ear. The electric potential is the source of energy for the sensory cells. See fig. 3.1. This is very expedient, since pulsating vessels close to the sensory organs would produce a disturbing noise.

The basis of the function of the sensory organs of the inner ear (including the sound transmitting cochlea) is a highly specialized cell, *the hair cell*, see fig. 3.3 below.

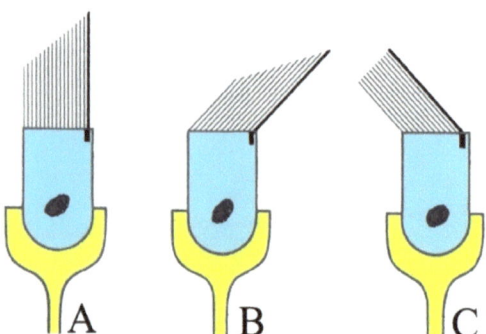

*Figure 3.3. The individual hair cells consist of a cell body and its hairs protruding into a gelatinous mass. There are two kinds of hair on each cell, one single thicker strand of hair, the **kinocilium,** and a number of thinner strands, the **sterocilia**. At rest (A), there is a constant discharge of nerve impulses from each cell.*

If physical forces result in a bending of the hairs, the cells produce a direction specific response: an increased firing rate in the nerve if the stimulus bend the hairs in the direction of the kinocilium (B) and a reduced response when bent in the opposite direction (C).

3.2.1 The **otolith organs**, (the **saccule** and the **utricle**)
The saccule and the utricle are both saclike structures containing endolymph. Covering part of their inner surface, there is a slightly cup-shaped plate, the sensory organs (*macula*) containing a large number of hair cells organized in a pattern that make the organs sensitive to gravitational pull and linear accelerations. In the case of the utricle, the sensory organ is mostly horizontal, for the saccule, the position is almost vertical.

The sensory cells, with their kinocilia of the four otolith organs, are arranged in a polarity pattern that makes the four organs together sensitive to gravity in any direction. Together, the four organs of the right and left ear essentially cover the surface of a small globe, providing useful and important information of the direction of the gravitational pull to the balance centers of the brain.

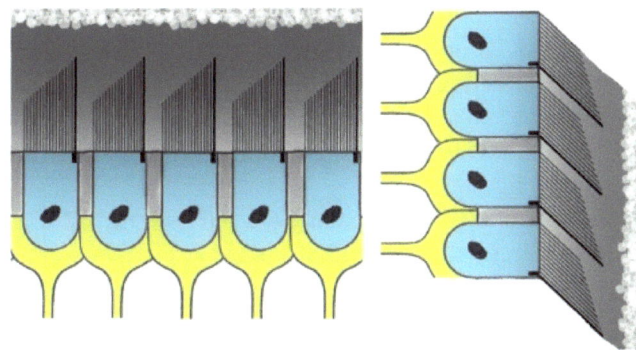

*Figure 3.4. The arrangement of the hair cells in the maculae of the otolith organs. The hair cells protrude into a gelatinous mass that becomes more and more viscous the farther it is from cell surface. The gelatinous mass is loaded with a membrane of small calcium crystals, the **otoconia**. A sliding motion of the membrane results in a deflection of the hairs (the right part of the figure).*

The primary mission of the otolith organs is to provide the brain with information about what is up and down, to make it possible for an individual to maintain balance, i.e. to make sure that the vertical projection of one's center of mass is a point within the base of support. This is a static description with reference only to a standing position, see fig. 3.5.

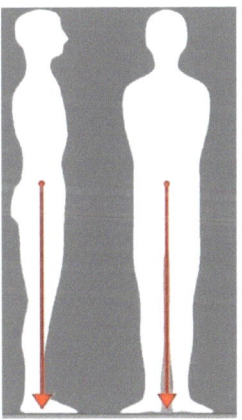

Figure 3.5. Balance when standing depends on the condition where the vertical projection of the person's center of gravity is found within an area determined by a person's feet.

Because of the anatomy of the feet, there is a tolerance of approximately 12° for forward leans and 5° for backward leans before a fall occurs. This refers to a non-physiological invert pendulum balance model (see fig 3.6 B). In real life, forward-backward sways are handled by a three-joint movement, (called "hip strategy") which involves opposite bending in the ankles, hips and the root of the neck, see fig. 3.6 C.

Lateral leans are handled by spreading the feet, see fig. 3.6 D. At the same time, the procedure facilitates the venous pump, or in other words shifting weight from one leg to the other induces muscular contractions in the opposite leg which forces the venous blood in the legs in the direction of the heart, as the venous valves only permit a flow of blood in that direction.

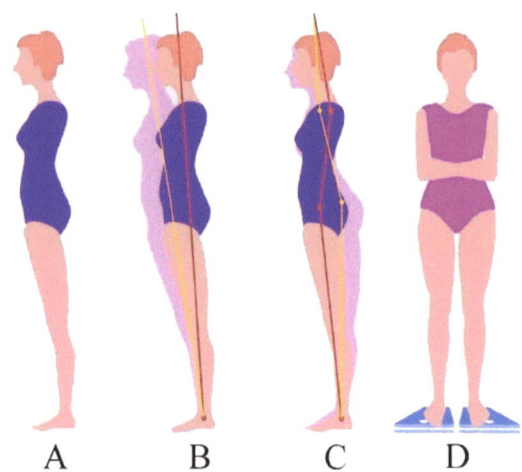

A B C D

Figure 3.6. Balance strategies, see text above for an explanation.

The task is much more complex when describing how the vertical projection point of the center of mass behaves and must behave during walk and run. For each step, when walking, this point must move from one supporting foot to the next. When running (which can be explained as a series of aborted forward falls) the point shows a serpent like figure between the footprints without touching them.

3.2.2 The semicircular canals
Both inner ears house three semicircular canals, each of which is perpendicular to the two other canals. The three-dimensional architecture ensures that all head motions around any axis of the head will be sensed by the

canals. The brain is trained to interpret the signals from the six canals to determine both the direction and the angular velocity of the head motion. Head motions appear as voluntary movements, as involuntary reflex movements, and as result of passive motions during locomotion. When walking and running, the head oscillates vertically in time with every step taken. This calls for opposite eye movements to compensate for head movement, to ensure a stable gaze direction. This canal reflex is named **the vestibulo-ocular reflex** (see fig 3.8). The way it works is that the head oscillations provoke an inertial reaction of the endolymph in the canals. This reaction is picked up by the sense organs of the canals the *ampular organs*, see fig. 3.7 below.

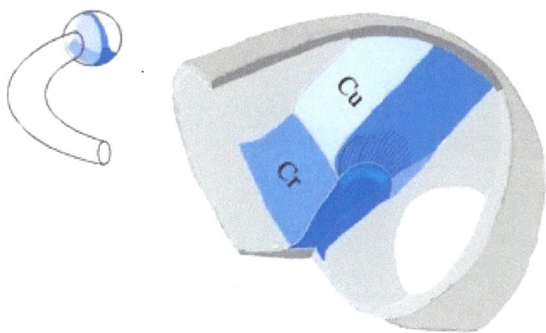

*Figure 3.7. The ampular sense organ of a semicircular canal. When the endolymph in the canal is under the influence of inertial forces caused by a movement of the head, a suction or a pull on soft structure in the ampulla occurs. This results in a stimulation of the hair cells of the organ. The dark blue firm base of the organ, the **crista** (Cr), houses a large number of sensory cells, their cilia protruding into the soft gelatinous mass of the light blue **cupula** (Cu) found above the crista. This stimulation produces a nerve signal, telling the brain about the direction and power of the movement.*

If constantly stimulated for more than a few seconds, the response in the ampular nerves fades out and in the end signals "no motion". In fact, during a constant rotation maintained for a certain amount of time, there will be no inertial forces either. This shows that the semicircular canals are fit for signaling relatively high frequency to-and-fro and up-down motions and not typically slow oscillations during transportation or constant rotations as in a fairground carousel. If suddenly terminating a slow frequency rotation, initial forces in the canals induce an unpleasant counter directional response if the individual is deprived of vision during the rotation. This is a most confusing dizzy experience often provoking an acute need of support.

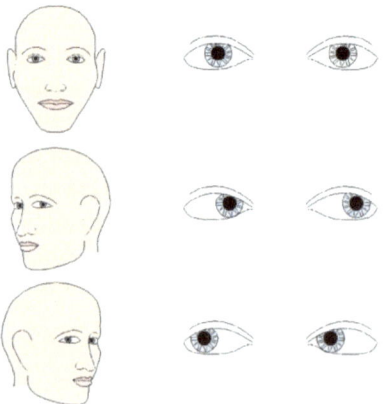

*Figure 3.8. The **vestibulo-ocular reflex (VOR)**. When the head turns to the right, the eyes turn to the left, and vice versa. This ensures a stable direction of vision during head motion.*

Under normal conditions, head movements are made at a relatively high frequency. A short head movement to the right will induce a biphasic perilymphatic splash-like pressure/suction to the ampular organ, as seen in fig. 3.9 below.

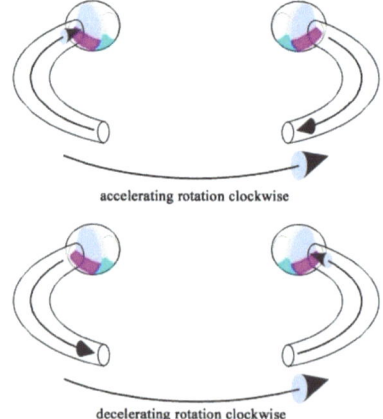

accelerating rotation clockwise

decelerating rotation clockwise

Figure 3.9. The canal response to a short head motion consisting of a short acceleration followed by a short deceleration of the head. The biphasic clockwise end-organ stimulus will result in a monophasic counter-clockwise eye movement response.

16

In order to achieve a perfect result, the vestibulo-ocular reflex (VOR) must be precise in time and amplitude. This is a learned response with a high degree of plasticity. If you have your eye glasses prescription changed, it will change the magnification effects of the lenses, calling for an amplitude adjustment of the vestibulo-ocular reflex. Usually people experience a few days of discomfort until they adapt to the new lenses. Following this, they will have two programs of different eye gains of the reflex at their disposal, one for glasses on, and one for glasses off. For people with a very myopic eyesight, who typically experience a very substantial change of magnification when changing between contact lenses and glasses, the adaptation usually works perfectly.

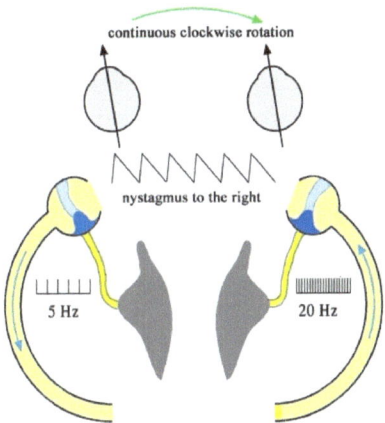

Figure 3.10. The principles of the vestibular nystagmus illustrated as a result of a continuous clockwise horizontal rotation. It appears from the figure (left canal) that suction on the ampular organ results in a reduction of the firing rate in the nerve. A pull on the organ will result in an increased firing rate.

3.3 Other physiologic functions related to balance function.

3.3.1 Visually induced eye movements
Eye movements caused by semicircular canal stimuli will be modified by two different types of more or less conscious eye movements:
1. Sudden changes in the direction of the gaze (**saccades**) caused by the incentive to bring an object sensed in the peripheral (or ambient) visual field or by directional hearing into attention *by placing it in the central (or focal) visual area* for identification. Saccades are extremely fast eye movements. They appear also in the form of the fast phases of vestibular nystagmus, as described above.

17

2. **Smooth pursuit** eye movements that appear when there is a need to retain a moving object in the central, focal visual field see fig. 3.12.

Some rather complex eye movement emerge when mixing the vestibulo-ocular responses (VOR) with saccades or/and smooth pursuit eye movement. This is very expedient because the function of saccades and smooth pursuit eye movements must be maintained during head movements

The smooth pursuit reflex makes it possible to maintain an object in the focal visual area of the retina. This means that it becomes possible to both identify and track the object. In humans, the pursuit reflex has developed into such an advanced function that the eyes are a little ahead of the object if the trajectory is known and recognized. If the object is a game animal, for example, a skilled hunter is able by reflex to locate the cross point between the two trajectories, that of the prey and that of his bullet, arrow, javelin, or rock.

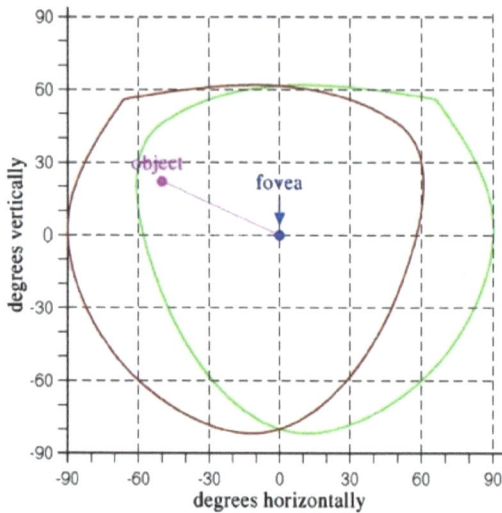

Figure 3.11. Visual field. Saccades are eye movements that bring objects from the peripheral visual field into central visual area (fovea).

Even for an average tennis player, this means that in a split second, based on the opponent's grip on the racket, the way the racket hits the ball, and an estimate of the force of the stroke, it is possible for the player to estimate the ball's trajectory, where and how to intercept the trajectory, or in the worst case establish the point of the final second impact on the surface of the court. Everything, whether it is an animal or a ball game, is usually performed during a continuous motion of the player.

18

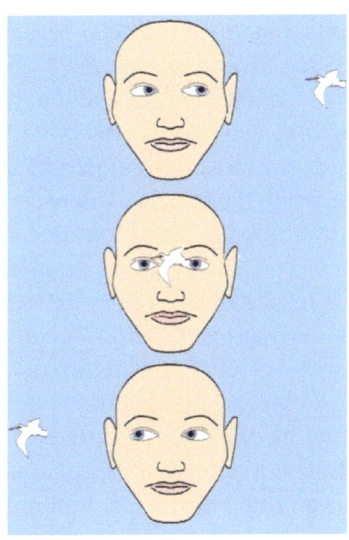

Figure 3.12. The smooth pursuit reflex. The eyes are able precisely to track a flying object.

3.3.2 Proprioception (and kinesthesia).

Proprioception is the sense of the relative position of different parts of the body. It depends on information from specialized sensors in muscles, tendons, and in the capsules of the joints. The information provided is used to monitor position as well as motion (kinesthesia). Motion is triggered by a more or less conscious intention to move from one position/location to another. This starts a series of neural activities influenced by experience and ends up in a **motor command** from the brain to relevant groups of muscles. Experience is a product of the past and contains the individual's strategies to deal with gravitation and navigation. The proprioceptive feedback, combined with sensory feedback from the inner ears, vision, and other senses, either confirms the efficacy of the muscular activation processes or gives rise to a change of the stored information on the muscle activation process because the motion was not that successful. The degree of complexity of the task is very high – the actual direction of gravitation must be considered in almost any motion. A certain group of muscles along the head-trunk-leg axis counteracts the gravitational pull in any upright position. At the same time, these muscles, as any other muscles, play their part in the locomotion process. Information of the exact direction of the gravitational pull is vital in this process.

3.3.3 Vision and hearing

In contrast to proprioception and the vestibular senses, both vision and hearing are occupied with what is happening *outside the body*.

Vision has two dimensions, the **central, focal or foveal vision** and the **peripheral or ambient vision,** which relies on two different, specialized types of sensory cells, cones and rods. The central part of the retina, the **fovea** (see fig. 3.11), is free of rods, while the cones are densely packed in the fovea. Foveal vision is highly developed in man (compare the smooth pursuit reflex above). Its function is to help identify objects by identifying colors, shapes, and motion patterns. It is responsible for the visual acuity, as tested by opticians and physicians. The peripheral or ambient vision originates from rods in the peripheral retina. Its function is to provide information about the coordinates of unspecified objects outside the fovea, to provoke saccades for the foveal identification of the objects, and further to provide a rough, easily disturbed, impression of the horizontal and vertical planes.

Directional hearing is an often neglected dimension of hearing. Just as a test of vision in most cases is a test of visual acuity, hearing tests as a principle are concerned with identifying thresholds of tones and word identification. Threshold detection is not the working field of the hearing in our daily life. Directional hearing identifies the direction to sources of sound. In humans and animals, it is a very precise function. Imagine a situation in which an animal cannot get a clear impression of the direction of a sound source coming from a friend or a foe; this animal will not survive for very long. The same situation will cause problems for humans, both in social situations and in traffic. This is the main complaint of patients who have suddenly lost hearing in one ear.

Together, ambient vision and directional hearing provide information about coordinates of the ambient world; focal vision and hearing informs us about the character of objects and individuals.

3.3.4 The central nervous system

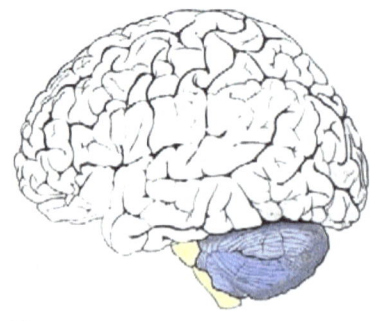

Figure 3.13. The brain. The cerebrum (white), the cerebellum (blue) and the brain stem (yellow).

The brain is a great and indispensable conductor of all bodily functions. It consists of the cerebrum, the cerebellum (the small brain), and the brain stem connecting to the spinal cord (see fig. 3.13). Together, including the spinal cord, it is named the **central nervous system**, the **CNS** among connoisseurs.

If the sensing of a physical event, i.e. the turn of the head, is going to have any consequence for an individual, e.g., resulting in a compensatory eye movement (the vestibulo-ocular reflex), information from the semicircular canal and proprioceptors in the muscles of the neck must be coupled to the part of the CNS responsible for eye movements. The connection takes place in the brain stem, in the central nuclei of the vestibular system. This is not to be compared with electric wiring, which connects the power plant with an electric bulb. The connection involves a large network of nerve cells for the interpretation of the sensory input and for the modification and fine tuning of the motor response, making use of a large portion of stored experience. The network does not only involve one specific part of the brain, but large, widely dispersed parts of the brain stem, the cerebellum and the cerebrum.

Humans developed from quadrupeds into bipeds thousands of years ago. At birth, unlike most quadruped animals, we have no control of our balance. It is a much more difficult task to move around on two legs compared to four. Locomotion on the hind legs must be taught during infancy. At first, we learn to maintain balance for a few seconds, supported by our parents or from furniture or other structures around us. Then one or two steps followed by a fall will be followed by more steps, eventually walking without support. During this first period, an infant is constantly at risk of falling or stumbling over any obstacle. Then as time passes, running and jumping is learned. The process might be described as "learning not to fall". Our locomotion has been described as a "symphony of mechanical and computational efficiency". Scientist struggle to reconstruct this when they construct walking robots.

Over the course of a lifetime, everybody at any time runs the risk of falling or stumbling, and might do so now and then. The fact is that a very large majority, thousands of falls, are avoided by the same reflex "how to avoid a fall", which might be named the ***anti-stumbling reflex***. A foot is moved in the direction of which the projection of the center mass moves – and voilà – balance is reestablished! A satisfactory function of the reflex turns walking and running into "the art of moving without falls". As we age, reflexes become slower and the muscle force necessary to prevent falls slowly diminish; as a consequence, the risk of falling increases, further advanced by impaired vision, which makes it difficult to see obstacles on the ground. Running skills disappear simultaneously with ageing, for *what is running but a series of consecutive falls aborted by the anti-stumbling reflex?*

3.3.6 A systems concept of balance

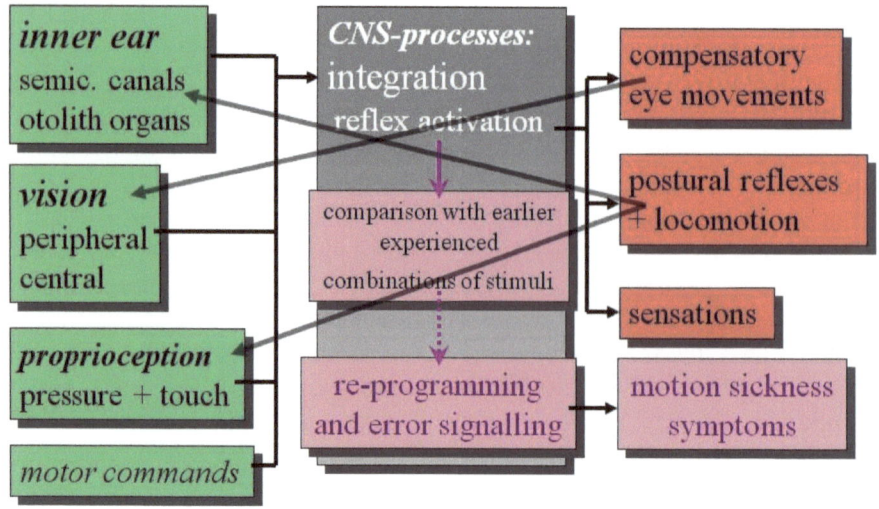

Figure 3.14. Flow of the balance system.

We call it a balance *system*, because the physiologic entities described above depend on each other and the function as a whole is more than the sum of the different particular functions. In any concept, the word *system* means something more advanced than its sum of partial elements. One reason for that is that it involves feedback control and an ability to adjust the procedures according to any inconvenient output result. Moving the eyes alters vision. Moving the body or body parts alter proprioception and stimulates the vestibular sense organs if the head moves as part of the movement, as sketched in fig. 3.14 above.

Then, which sensory function is the most important for the balance? It seems that the vestibular input from the semicircular canals and otolith organs plays a major role in balance, because a sudden loss of these functions in one or both inner ears is a major disaster for balance.

Loss of proprioception is disastrous too. Imagine for yourself that because of crossing your legs in a sitting position, one of your legs goes to sleep. If you rise, it will impossible to maintain balance and you will immediately seek support. Both cases, loss of vestibular function and loss of proprioception and pressure sense from the soles of the feet are much worse for balance compared to e.g. a sudden loss of vision.

It appears from fig. 3.14 that a re-programming of the system may take place if a comparison of earlier and actual stimulus combination results in a deficit of appropriateness of the output. If bad enough, the price can be an error signal leading to motion sickness symptoms. This is an enigma not yet solved. One of very few, if any, reactions in the CNS that is so inappropriate, and more than a century of research has produced no clues whatsoever of why or how.

Motion sickness is a major inconvenience when traveling, especially at sea. It is a major risk factor for an aggressor when moving troops from their original location to a battle field and it is a security factor during the first days of space missions. Those who suffer from motion sickness are not very efficient individuals and some may even as part of their motion sickness symptoms become so mentally depressed that they may become suicidal. Such individuals do not make very good soldiers and are expensive, inefficient astronauts (not to mention that they, if incautious, would have to live/work with their roommates in a space craft contaminated by free floating vomit). Motion sickness is one of a number of good reasons not to start a war, but it should not prevent us from traveling the world or exploring space. It seems that the vestibular input from the semicircular canals and otolith organs plays a major role in balance, because a sudden loss of these functions in one or both inner ears is a major disaster for balance. Loss of proprioception is disastrous too, as mentioned above.

It appears from fig. 3.14 that a re-programming of the system may take place if a comparison of earlier and actual stimulus combination results in a deficit of appropriateness of the output. If bad enough, the price can be an error signal leading to motion sickness symptoms. This is an enigma not yet solved. One of very few, if any, reactions in the CNS that is so inappropriate that more than a century of research has produced no clues whatsoever of why or how.

Motion sickness is a major inconvenience when traveling, especially at sea. It is a major risk factor for an aggressor when moving troops from their original location to a battle field and a security factor during the first days of space missions. Those who suffer from motion sickness are not very efficient individuals and some may even as part of their motion sickness symptoms become so depressed that they may become suicidal. Such individuals do not make very good soldiers and are expensive, inefficient astronauts (not to mention they would have to live/work in a space craft contaminated by free floating vomit). Motion sickness is one of a number of good reasons not to start a war, but should not prevent us from traveling the world's end or exploring space.

4. THE CONCEPT OF DIZZINESS AND VERTIGO

The vocabulary used by patients suffering from dysfunction of their balance systems varies a great deal.

Words like *whirling* or *dazed sensations*, *giddiness*, *lightheadedness*, *confusion,* or *bewilderment* are used to describe the symptoms. They are more or less specific or not very comprehensible. *Vertigo* is a more specific term covering a feeling of being spun around or that the surroundings are spinning around oneself. Vertigo is more firmly connected with a specific spinning movement than the word dizziness and relates more to the symptoms appearing when there is a loss of the vestibular sense of the inner ear, especially that of the semicircular canal function.

Closely related to balance function are our more or less conscious experience with the surrounding world, our *spatial orientation*. This concerns not only the experience of what is up and down and/or what is moving and what is not moving, but being a broader experience of qualities and quantities of the surrounding world, which, when disturbed, leads to *disorientation*. Dizziness and vertigo include disorientation and psychological complications that include mental depression, a symptom prominent in motion sickness.

The more specific and vertigo-like the symptoms are, the more likely it is that the patient also suffers from very unpleasant motion sickness symptoms like nausea and vomiting accompanying the dizziness and vertigo symptoms.

Being *unsteady*, *unbalanced,* or *losing balance* always accompanies dizziness. It is important that these symptoms may appear as independent phenomena. In these cases, disorders affecting the CNS, the nerves, or the locomotion apparatus must be considered, or conditions specifically affecting the otolith organs without involving the semicircular canals.

4.1 Concomitant symptoms

Dizziness or vertigo appearing simultaneously with *aural symptoms* such as hearing deterioration, hearing distortion, tinnitus, and/or aural fullness strongly indicate an ear disorder, usually inner ear problems.

Lightheadedness with a *sensation of fainting* suggest troubles with maintaining a sufficient blood pressure, constitutional of nature or caused by a heart problem or a neurologic disorder.

Accompanying neurological symptoms, such as areas of numbness, alteration in muscular force, speech problems, a sensation of brain fog, or any other symptom not directly related to dizziness, may indicate neurologic disorders and a need for an evaluation by a neurologist.

5. NATURES OF THE VESTIBULAR DYSFUNCTIONS LEADING TO VERTIGO/DIZZINESS.

5.1 Loss of function

To most physicians, a partial or a total loss of the sensitivity in the vestibular senses is the universal explanation of the appearance of inner ear dizziness. That loss of function leads to a phenomenon very much alike stimulation is clearly contradictory, unless those claiming it are familiar with the detailed physiology of the canal system (compare p. 15, fig. 3.10 and fig. 5.1 below).

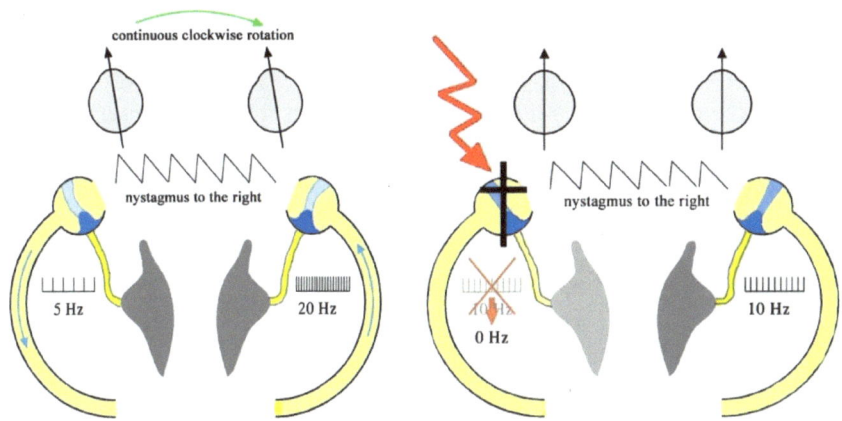

Figure 5.1. Left: a horizontal, clockwise rotation in the plane of the two horizontal semicircular canals will cause a nystagmus directed to the right, sometimes accompanied by a feeling of rotation to the right, depending on the magnitude of the rotational acceleration, the presence of visual orientation and on the focus of attention of the person, compare fig. 3.9. The polarization of the stimulus results in a decreasing firing rate of the left ampular nerve and an increasing firing in the right nerve. Right: in the case of a destruction of the function of the left canal, there will be no nerve signals from the left side and a normal resting signal in the right ampular nerve. In the brain this asymmetry of signals is interpreted as a clockwise rotation, and the patient will consequently experience a clockwise spinning and a right directed nystagmus can be observed.

The golden rule (with reference to fig. 5.1) is that:

a destructive unilateral inner ear disorder will lead to a spinning sensation and nystagmus, both phenomena in the opposite direction compared to the site of the destruction.

This is a clear exception to the rule that a destruction of an organ leads to signs and symptoms of loss of function. Often, the destruction of semicircular function will strike all three canals; nevertheless, nystagmus will become mostly horizontal, probably because of the fact that our normal locomotion is horizontal, two-dimensional limited to the surface of our planet.

Abolition of the otolith organ function follows the general rule of organ destruction symptoms. Signals from the otolith organs of the paralyzed side are lacking and missed by the brain, and physical balance suffers. So if the spinning sensation alone does not kill balance, the otolith organs will complete the job.

5.2 Inner ear hypersensitivity

Hypersensitivity of the canal system is seen in BPPV (see 7.4). In this case, it is caused by the presence of a lump of *otoconia* (se p. 41) from the *utricle* dislocated to the canal, either functioning as a free-floating piston in the canal driven by gravitation or in a few cases as a heavy load on the cupula of an ampular organ, making the organ sensitive to gravitation. This causes an amplification of the canal specific stimuli or a positional irrelevant stimulation of the ampular organ, respectively.

5.3 Variable sensitivity

Another, not uncommon type of hypersensitivity is found in inner ears that suffer from endolyphatic pressure increase and results in a dilatation condition as seen in *Menière's disease* and probably also in *migraine vertigo* (see 7.5 and 7.6). In these cases, the endolymphatic pressure alternates and episodes of hypersensitivity are succeeded by normal sensitivity or hyposensitivity, signaling that an attack of vertigo or dizziness accompanied by hypersensitivity to sounds, tinnitus and aural fullness has terminated. The brain has difficulties in compensating for frequent variability in sensory function, which leave these patients with uncompensated sensory problems.

6. TESTS OF THE BALANCE FUNCTION

By tradition, there are a number of more or less standardized clinical examination techniques usually performed in patients complaining of dizziness. Now, most of them should be replaced by laboratory tests of a much more specific and documented nature.

One of the most important new options is the possibility of obtaining clear and well documented information of the state of function of the otolith organs.

6.1 Semicircular canals

In the classic dizziness clinic, rule number one is to look for nystagmus. If the patient is able visually to fixate, it is possible for the patient to suppress the nystagmus. One way to circumvent that problem is to have the patients close their eyes. If there is a nystagmus, it is possible to see that something is happening behind the eyelids, but to really see exactly what is happening is impossible.

There are two possible solutions to that problem. The first is to observe the nystagmus when the patient looks straight forward, then with the gaze to one side, followed by a gaze in the opposite direction. Nystagmus may be observed with patient's gaze in one, two or all three directions, making use of what is called **Alexander's law**. If present only in one direction, the direction of the nystagmus is in the direction of the gaze. This is called *Alexander grade 1*. When present in two directions – straight forward and in the gaze direction according the nystagmus, it is termed *Alexander grade 2,* and present in all gaze direction it is indeed *grade 3* nystagmus. It is an easy, un-instrumented, but unfortunately not very sensitive way of bedside evaluation of visible nystagmus, without the use of any aids, see fig. 6.1.

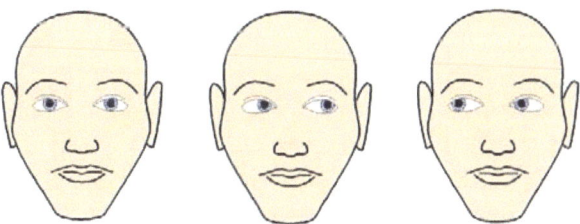

Figure 6.1 Alexander's law, see text above.

In most cases, the examiner will need an instrument to prevent the suppression of the nystagmus caused by visual fixation. The simplest device is a pair of goggles, known as Frenzel's goggles, see fig. 6.2, next page.

27

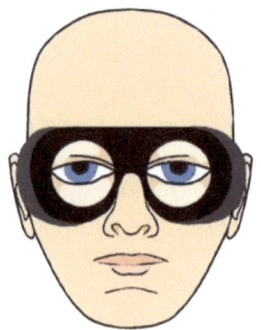

Figure 6.2. Frenzel's goggles. 15 diopter bi-convex lenses blur the patient's vision and magnifies the eyes so that the examiner more easily can observe the nystagmus or any other eye movements. There is a built-in illumination that further facilitates observation.

Using Frenzel's goggles is simple when observing nystagmus with the patient sitting in an upright position. It becomes more difficult if the task is to see if there is nystagmus in the supine position and when lying on the left or right side. It takes a great deal of effort and bending for the examiner to get around the patient. However, it is important to do so, because certain types of nystagmus (positio*nal* nystagmus) are only present in specific positions or following certain head movements (positio*ning* nystagmus).

The problem of diagnosing an observed nystagmus directly is that the presence of nystagmus is very sensitive to the patient's level of alertness. If the patient is tired and sleepy, the nystagmus may be obvious; if awake and alert, it might be gone. Another problem is that, except for Alexander's rather uncertain classification, it is difficult to grade the nystagmus. It is relatively easy to observe the direction of the nystagmus (in very forceful nystagmus, where the slow phase velocity may be close to the fast phase velocity, and it may be difficult to distinguish the two phase).

The solution to this is to let video cameras do the job. Using a high frame video frequency, feeding the signal to a computer to print the eye movements and to calculate how vigorous the present nystagmus is. The result can be stored and compared to nystagmus of other patients or the progress or any other change can be monitored for individual patients. The patient has to visit a laboratory, which most patients must do anyway. The technique is named VideoNystagmoGraphy (VNG). As mentioned below, a number of other meaningful tests may be performed in the lab at the same occasion.

This was about the very important phenomenon of pathologic nystagmus, but nothing about tests demonstrating if the canals work or to which degree they function. The classic and most used test of functional deficiencies of the semicircular canals is based on a strange phenomenon known as the **caloric**

28

reaction. This is not a part of what may be considered as a meaningful physiology of the inner ear. If one ear canal is irrigated with water of a temperature different from body temperature, a normal person will develop vertigo and horizontal nystagmus, provided that the patient's horizontal semicircular canal is in a vertical or near-vertical position. If the temperature of the water is below body temperature, the nystagmus and turning sensation of the patient will be in the opposite direction (as in a paralysis of the canal); if the temperature is above body temperature, the opposite will happen. The advantage of this test is that it is possible to test each ear separately and get a figure describing the functional state of that particular horizontal canal, which can be compared with the values obtained from the opposite ear. The nystagmus is easily recorded by means of VNG. The slow phase velocity of the nystagmus is considered the most reliable parameter, and it is easily calculated by computers. *There are, however, a number serious drawbacks when using caloric tests.* Only the horizontal canal is tested. The worst is that the brain knows that something strange and very un-physiological is going on. "Why is one ear spinning around and the other ear is not?" - "Why are my other senses, including my common sense, telling me that I'm lying still on my back?" The brain will start fighting back, and the efficiency of the fight depends on the alertness and fighting capacity of the person. The brain will start producing error signals resulting in motion sickness symptoms like nausea, and some dizzy patients will resign to their fate *"I came here dizzy, now it is worse, what can I expect from my disease and my doctor? Should I be seeing a doctor with a little more empathy?"*. Still, the caloric test even unpleasant and unprecise is the most commonly used test to evaluate canal function.

Another option is to make use of a *natural canal stimulus*. It is not as unpleasant for the patient as the caloric tests, and in most cases more informative, even when talking about differentiating between disorders of the left and the right ear. By nature, the canal responses are linked to high frequency stimuli, which means that slow head movements are picked up by vision and compensatory eye movements are produced by smooth pursuit like reactions. At higher frequencies vision becomes insufficient, and the canals take over because the vestibulo-ocular reflex preferably works at frequencies where vision is incapable of catching up.

The simplest clinical test is the **head-shaking test**. Shake the patient's head relatively quickly for a while, left-right-left-right etc., with the patient's eyes closed. If there is a functional weakness of the left horizontal canal, the signal to the brain will become "less rotation to the left, more rotation to the right" – the result being a net rotation to the right calling for a rightward horizontal nystagmus and rotational feeling. When the patients open their eyes, you will see a horizontal nystagmus to the right. If this test is performed with a simultaneous recording of head and eye movements, a computerized calculation of the transfer function between head and eye movements, it becomes a meaningful laboratory test. A *transfer function* is a mathematical expression of what should be done to the input signal (head oscillations) to make it identical with the output signal (eye movements). Question no. one: should it be subdued or amplified? The parameter is called the *output gain*. Question no. two is: is it synchronous? The parameter describing this is called the *phase deviation*. The computation is done using a what is known as a fast Fourier transformation and the result refers to gains and phase deviations at different frequencies of head shaking, not in time order of the events. When responding to these relatively forceful head movements, compensation of function deficiencies seems to be less pronounced at higher frequencies, compared to lower frequencies in accordance with patients' reaction to canal deficiencies – patients typically move much slower than before they became sick. Compensation of hyposensitivity is first seen in the phase (timing) parameter, probably because untimely eye responses are more disturbing than reductions of the size (amplitude) of the eye movements compared to the head movements. In my opinion, this test, known as the **Vestibular Autorotation Test®,** is much more meaningful than other vestibular tests aimed at the canal function, because it describes both reduction and hypersensitivity phenomena of the function and to some degree works independently of compensation, at least at higher frequencies. Asymmetries are revealed by directional preponderances as in the original head shaking test.

Another approach to the canals is to produce impulse stimuli and recording the compensatory eye responses, either by observing eye movement directly or by recording head and eye movements simultaneously. This is called the ***head impulse test*** (HIT). Recorded by means of fast video cameras it is v-HIT. It can be performed for all six canals, but the plain daily test is targeting the horizontal canal alone. Because of the asymmetry in modifying the firing rate in the ampular nerves (compare fig. 3.10), reduction of firing rates has a much lesser dynamic range (easily going towards zero) than increasing firing rate and the test has a sufficiently high ability to distinguish between right and left disturbances. The normal eye response mirrors the head movement as seen in fig. 6.3. With the results that follows a paralysis of one side, there is still a low gain response in the paralyzed direction, originating from the normal ear. A paralysis of one canal function shows up as a reduction of the amplitude of the eye movements compared to the head movement, but the shape of the two curves are very much alike.

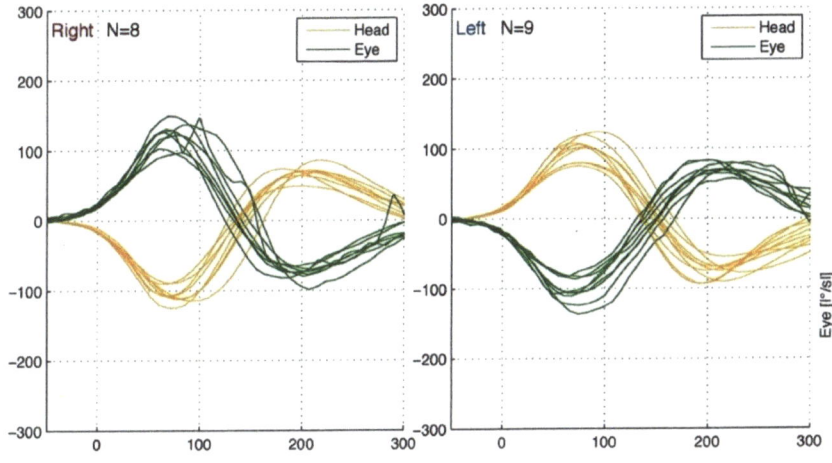

Figure 6.3. A normal response of a v-HIT, right and left side at a horizontal video impulse test (v-HIT).

Compensation for a reduced or abolished function appears very soon after the event in the form of saccades filling out the need of a sufficient gain. In the first instance, the compensatory saccades appear later than the immediate response; afterward it will come earlier and earlier and by that compensate more sufficiently time-wise for the paralysis. A normal response is seen in fig. 6.3 above.

6.2 Otolith organs.

Otolith organ information about the direction of the gravitational pull is vital to our general orientation and locomotion, and compensatory measures are lined up, if the otolith organs fail to work. This explains why observing a dizzy patient standing upright or walking is no guarantee of a normal otolith function.

Vision is first in line to induce some compensation. Proprioception, pressure, and touch sensing are next to compensate. The classic test for this is the Romberg test (see fig. 6.4). In this test, the patient is told to stand eyes closed, feet together, arms crossed, and the examiner observes if there are any sways judged to be abnormal; if positive, is there a predominant direction of the sways? Normal people easily pass the test, even though some sway appears in normal people when their eyes are closed. So the question is: is the performance normal? Older people tend to sway more than younger people when their eyes are closed. If the test is "very" positive, the patient may fall

31

the instant they close their eyes. We can make it a little more difficult for the patient by having the patient observe a tandem position, "heel against toes". Some normal people will fall just because they are deprived of the opportunity to spread their legs.

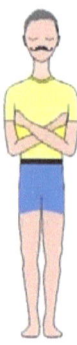

Figure 6.4. The Romberg test, patient standing eyes closed, feet together and arms crossed.

Romberg's test may be performed in a more advanced way by using three different visual conditions: 1. eyes open, 2. blindfolded and 3. with a stable visual field, uninfluenced by head motions by means of a small lightweight dome; it is named the *sensory organization test*. The patient may stand on the floor or on a compliant surface such as a foam rubber mat. This version is called the *Clinical Test for Sensory Interaction in Balance (CTSIB)*, see fig. 6.5. The same procedure can be performed by means of a computerized force platform setup, then named a *computerized dynamic posturography*.

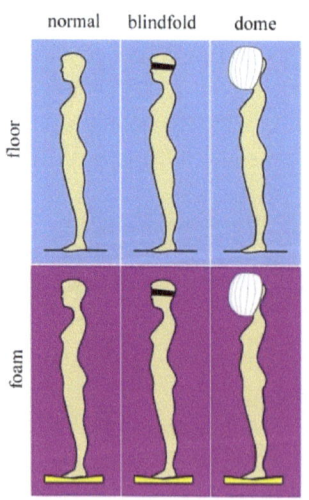

Figure 6.5. The CTSIB test and its six different conditions. The dome procedure is not used often, but the other four conditions have proven valuable. Time to near-fall is the parameter used. The examiner must be ready to prevent possible falls.

Tests of balance of this type have proven valuable for the follow-up of patients, e.g., those who have had vestibular rehabilitation therapy. However, they are not very meaningful in the context of individual etiological diagnostics.

The last 15-20 years have provided us with much more meaningful and specific test methods for the function of the otolith organs. It has been known for a relatively long time that the otolith organs can be stimulated by short and loud sounds. The stimulation will in the case of saccule result in a short, approximately 10 ms (milliseconds) relaxation of muscles around the longitudinal axis, those counteracting the gravitational pull, or of the eye muscles in the case of stimulating the utricle. The test procedures are termed "Vestibular Evoked Potential" tests, VEMP. *cVEMP* (c for cervical) tests the *saccule* on the same side as the sound stimulus, typically presented as a number of very short clicks at a relatively high loudness (e.g., 95dB as demonstrated in fig. 6.6 below). The relatively high volume of the sound stimuli is unproblematic because of the very short duration of the clicks (typically 0.1 ms).

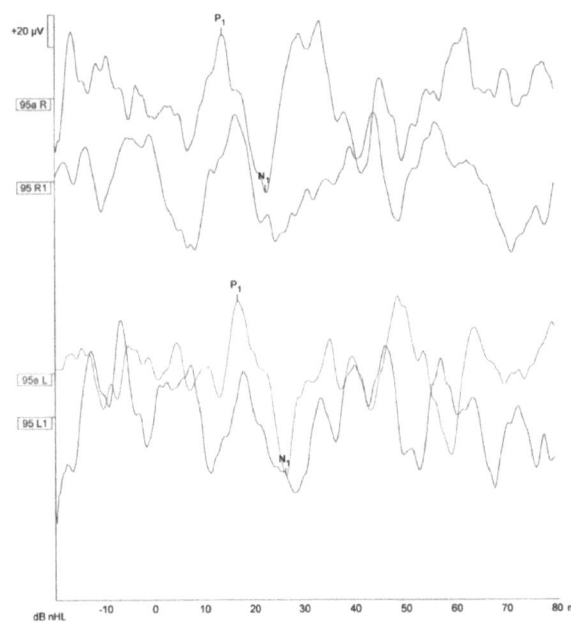

Figure 6.6. cVEMP responses from a normal person obtained by recording surface EMGs (ElectroMyoGraphy) from the sternocleidomastoidal muscle (the thick muscle on each side of the front of the neck). Red curves are the right ear -- blue curves are the left ear.

oVEMPs (o for ocular) are produced using a similar protocol but record from muscles around the eye ball, using surface electrodes placed above and below the orbit on the other side of the ear stimulated or by stimulating with a tuning fork or a tap in the midline of the top of the head. oVEMPs describe the function of the *utricle*.

The VEMP methods have had a very important impact on the understanding of otolith organ dysfunction. Typically, patients suffering from otolith dysfunctions only present with a confusing symptomatology, like feeling uncertain of what is up and down, with lightheadedness or giddiness, very often interpreted as originating from a psychological dysfunction rather than a somatic origin. It has been a lesson learned that unknown etiology (the cause of a disease) is not equivalent to psychogenic disorder.

6.3 Other test procedures

Both saccades and smooth pursuit eye movements should be tested in order to be informed about other functions relevant to the balance system and sensitive to pathology in the brainstem and the cerebellum, see fig. 6.7. The video recording technique (VNG) is very useful for this purpose, too.

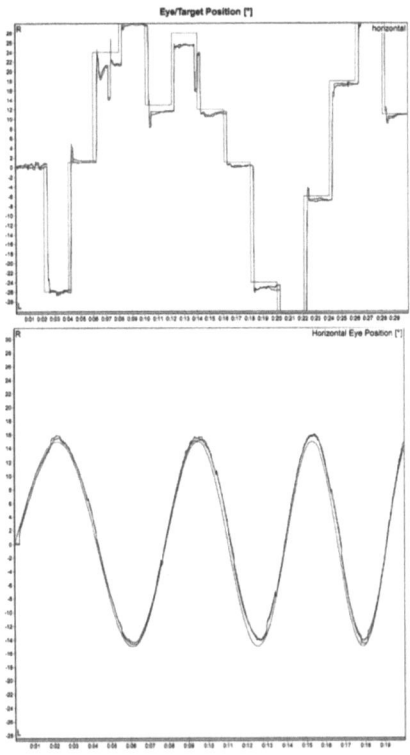

Figure 6.7. Tests of saccades (above) and smooth pursuit eye movements (below), showing normal responses.

In all cases, *hearing tests* should be performed to rule out any hearing abnormalities, even in cases where the patient has no hearing complaints. Even small differences between the right and left ears should be pursued to make certain hearing differences are diagnosed by their cause.

Brain scans should be performed under two different indications:

1. There is reason to suspect CNS pathology because of symptoms or abnormal test results unrelated to the vestibular system.
2. The patient is concerned that they have a serious CNS disease.

Neither CAT- nor MRI-scans provide useful details of the inner ear. If for some reason there for is suspicion of an acoustic neuroma (vestibular schwannoma), an MRI-scan is indicated.

Methods are developing that will compensate for the inability of the MRI-scans to visualize the inner ear, and a few clinics offer these sensitive technologies. Whether such techniques will replace meticulous function diagnostics is questionable, but they might provide a useful supplement to test of balance function.

It is worthwhile keeping in mind that patients usually do not complain of an abnormal *appearance* of the inner ear or the brain, but complain of functional disturbances. Seeing such disturbances in test results facilitates the doctor's understanding of the patient's story and complaints, and makes it possible to follow-up on treatment results or spontaneous improvement.

Test results are unsurpassed as a means of communication between doctor and patient because there is a high degree of correlation between test results and patient complaints. It helps a great deal that the methods have grown much more relevant, reliable, specific, and sensitive.

Images are made for surgeons and they are a great help when planning and understanding surgery. Physiology is for the internists.

7. DISEASES CAUSING DIZZINESS AND VERTIGO

7.1 A key to the diagnosis of some types of dizziness and vertigo.

Duration of attack	Type of dizziness	Nature of vestibular dysfunction	Diagnosis
Symptoms wane in weeks or months	Continuous, vertigo-type Violent Spinning	Impairment	Vestibular Neuritis (see 7.3)
20-30 seconds	Violent Spinning-type Provoked by specific motions	Canal hypersensitivity	BPPV (see 7.4)
20 minutes to 12 hours	Violent Unprovoked Accompanied by hearing symptoms	Variable	Menière's disease (see 7.5)
From minutes to constant and fluctuating in strength	Moderate to strong Unbalanced Accompanied by headache and hearing symptoms	Variable	Migraine vertigo (see 7.6)
Varying depending on provocation	Short lasting Provoked by sounds or exercise or pressure Hearing deterioration	Hypersensitivity	Dehiscense syndrome (see 7.7.2)
Seconds to minutes Good days/bad days	Fainting and sensation of remoteness	No dysfunction	Low BP Fainting syndrome (see 7.8)
Most bothering during motion	Un-characteristic Bothersome during locomotion.Accompanied by non–acoustic neurological symptoms	?	CNS disease (see 7.9)

7.2 Vestibular neuritis

Vestibular neuritis is a dramatic disease that starts very suddenly in most patients. A sudden uneasy feeling accelerates in minutes into a feeling of maximal discomfort due to a violent, incapacitating, spinning sensation, soon accompanied by nausea, vomiting, and the loss the ability to stand on one's legs. Many patients and witnesses will suspect a cerebral stroke, but the only bodily function not working is the vestibular contribution to balance, in the worst case semicircular canals and otolith organs in one ear, all included.

The symptoms tell the story of the significance of the vestibular organs for balance and wellbeing. There are no other symptoms, no hearing disturbances and no signs of neurologic dysfunction such as loss of speech, numbness or other paralyses than that affecting the vestibular organs. From observing the patient's eyes, even behind closed eyelids, it is obvious that there is rigorous nystagmus.

The only immediate way to establish which ear is suffering is to determine the direction of the nystagmus. It will beat away from the suffering ear. In some cases, it is clear that the nystagmus is a *combination of a horizontally beating at the same time torsional eye movements,* which indicates that the lower branch of the balance nerve may not be involved in the disease. The lower branch carries signals from the saccule and the inferior canal. In some cases, when only the lower branch of the nerve is involved, the clinical picture is dominated by the loss of balance due to the involvement of the saccule combined with a paralyses of the inferior semicircular canal. So in the principle there are three different pictures, depending on which part or parts of the balance nerve are involved.

So what can be done for a very ill patient who everybody fears is having a cerebral stroke? Most patients will end up in an emergency room, hopefully encountering medical staff familiar with the diagnosis. After all it is the third most common cause of peripheral vertigo, with a prevalence of 3.5 per 10,000 inhabitants. It is more common in younger than in older members of the population. The clinical diagnosis is relatively easy, but it is important that a *cerebellar,* or a *small brainstem stroke,* is considered as the only, but also relative rare, differential diagnosis to vestibular neuritis.

The examination of the patient involves a study of the nystagmus, and most importantly also the simple *head impulse test,* see p. 30. The latter is very important because a nystagmus may also be present in patients suffering from a cerebellar stroke, but an abnormal response to the head impulse test is specific to the loss of inner ear canal function.

In cases where there is doubt about the cause of the symptoms, a brain scan must be performed. In cases presenting an abnormal impulse test, a scan study should at least be postponed. A patient with a violent vertigo, who prefers to lie down on their healthy side to achieve just a bit of comfort, should not be brought into a scanner, where a supine position and a demand to lie still is a precondition for a successful result. If there are no other clinical signs or symptoms indicating a CNS disorder, the patient will be better off without much ado.

There is evidence that a short, high dose steroid treatment will reduce the symptom load on the patient and shortening the very long, weeks or months, of disabling vertigo symptoms.

It is important to start a vestibular rehabilitation program by a physiotherapist as soon as possible. And it is important, too, to realize that a vestibular neuritis patient has very few resources to draw on. It is an energy consuming condition. It is absolutely counter-productive to prescribe sedatives, including vestibular sedatives (anti-motion sickness remedies). The duration of the period of rehabilitation is very age dependent. For young people it may be a number of weeks, for elderly people it is months. The rehabilitation program must include the consideration of loss of muscular fitness when a patient is immobilized by dizziness for such a period of time.

Many patients end up with a sensory deficit concerning vestibular function. Quite a large number of former neuritis patients will experience BPPV-attacks (see 7.4, p. 41) in the years following their neuritis. It is important that the patients are aware of this and know that it is possible to offer a much more efficient treatment of that condition. The symptoms of BPPV may mimic neuritis with violent spinning sensations, but differ by the fact that keeping still prevents the vertigo, that the duration of an attack is short, and that the vertigo attacks are provoked by certain well-defined head motions.

Some patients seem to stick with their dizziness due to anxiety of falling. They have attacks of short discomfort when confronted with specific situations. They experience a feeling very much like the feeling you get when climbing a ladder and stepping on a loose rung. While this lasts only seconds, it is accompanied by anxiety, a lump in the stomach and clammy hands. Explaining to the patient the mechanisms behind this is very often a sufficient treatment. The condition is known as *phobic postural vertigo* (see 7.11).

7.3 Other conditions caused by a loss of vestibular function
7.3.1 Inner ear dysfunction caused by head trauma
In the case of severe head traumas, the inner ear may suffer. In some case there is a fracture involving the petrous part of the temporal bone, a complex bony structure in the base of the skull. Fracture lines are, due to the complex structure, intricate and not easily seen on an X-ray or CAT-scan. If there are

38

signs of bleeding in the skin behind the ear and/or symptoms or signs of a blood-filled middle ear (as seen by otoscopy or on a CAT-scan), it is a clear indication of a fracture. If the fracture line involves the inner ear, the patient will usually suffer a severe hearing loss and signs and symptoms of vestibular paralysis, i.e. severe vertigo and nystagmus towards the opposite ear. The facial nerve, responsible for motions of the muscles of the face and for the taste on a large part of the tongue on the same side, may suffer because of its passage through a bony canal of the inner ear.

In some patients there may be another explanation of dizziness and hearing complaints following a blunt head trauma or a whip-lash trauma, a perilymphatic fistula (see 7.7.3), or in much more common and simple case, signs and symptoms of BPPV (see 7.4).

In the case of a *bilateral* lesion and the consequent bilateral abolition of vestibular function, the patient's prime complaint will be an extremely stressful loss of balance and to a lesser degree dizziness, which will only be present during locomotion, compare 7.3.2 below. In the worst cases there is a bilateral loss of hearing, and the patient will feel totally lost. It is important to institute a vestibular rehabilitation program as soon as the patient's condition allows.

7.3.2 Ototoxic lesions
A few medicaments may have a toxic effect on the inner ear. This is the case for the *aminoglycosides*, antibiotics used in order to fight infections very often of a life-threatening type, of which one of the most popular is *gentamicin*. Aminoglycosides have a tendency to accumulate in the inner ear and if their concentration in the inner ear fluids is above a certain level, they will cause an irreversible lesion to the inner ear, usually both ears, because the drug circulating in the bloodstream will be presented equally to both inner ears. Their blood concentration should be checked in all cases and it should be considered that patients suffering from kidney diseases tend to accumulate the drug in the blood putting the inner ears at risk. In toxic doses, the immediate consequence for the inner ear is a loss of hair cells, for gentamicin primary in the vestibular organs but also at higher concentrations in the cochlea, so not only balance function, but also hearing is under threat.

A *bilateral* vestibular lesion will show up much more as a loss of balance than as dizziness. There will be no nystagmus either. When on the feet, the patient is unable to maintain balance and walking is impossible without the support of another person. When walking, the spontaneous up and down motion of the head in time with the steps will cause the image of the world around to move up and down in time with the steps. This is called *oscilopsia*.

This phenomenon is seen only with a bilateral loss of the vestibulo-ocular reflex and contributes to the balance problems by causing *visual dizziness*. The very sad thing is that in these cases, the balance function will not return. In cases of ototoxic lesions, it is important to start vestibular rehabilitation as soon as the patient has recovered from the (often life-threatening) infection.

Lesions of this type are rare because of the availability of blood-testing of concentration of the aminoglycosides and the awareness of most healthcare staff to this specific adverse effect to that drug family.

7.3.3 Acoustic neuroma = vestibular schwannoma[1]

The clinical picture of this *100% benign tumor* has changed in time with the more and more refined techniques used with MRI-scans. It is now possible to diagnose tumors in the size of order of less than 1 mm (0.04 inches). With the increasing sensitivity of the method, smaller tumors are found and more tumors have been diagnosed.

Fortunately, at the same time, research has shown that some tumors do not grow anymore at the time of the diagnosis. This has led to a "wait-and-scan"-policy in the case of small tumors "only" harming hearing and balance. This is reasonable because treatment, surgery or irradiation, puts the balance function, the hearing, and facial motions at risk. So the price of treatment often is a deterioration of these functions to save the patient from the price of the growth of the tumor, which may not only lead to deterioration of hearing, balance, and facial motion but also to the risk of symptoms associated with a compression of the brainstem and cerebellum.

In most cases, balance studies show a deficit in balance nerve function, but in a majority of those cases, compensation has developed in time with the slowly progressing loss of function. This is another clinical demonstration of the capacity of brain recue of unilateral vestibular loss of function.

7.3.4 Idiopathic bilateral vestibulopathia[2]

This is a relatively rare condition, which shows up as a progressive loss of parts of or all or most vestibular sensory qualities. In its end stage, it can be compared with the ototoxic lesions, but patients have a chance to partially compensate during the development of ailment.

---

[1] Officially, the term *acoustic neuroma* has been replaced by vestibular schwannoma because benign tumors do not originate from nerve tissue of the acoustic nerve, but from the nerve sheaths of (in most cases) the adjacent vestibular nerve.

[2] *Idiopathic* means of unknown or uncertain origin, and not coming from nowhere its etymological meaning.

40

7.4 BPPV, Benign Paroxysmal Positional Vertigo.

BPPV accounts for approximately 30% of all visits to specialized dizziness clinics. It is the most common cause of vertigo, and in some contexts the most overlooked cause of vestibular dysfunction, especially when talking about the elderly population. To miss the diagnosis of a condition so relatively easily diagnosed and cured is a great shame. It is one of a few "sick man in - healthy man out" disorders. Maybe it is not easily learned, but it is a worthwhile effort for any physician at the risk of meeting dizzy patients to study the theory and practice of the art of diagnosing and treating this ailment.

Symptoms are very specific and in most cases easily recognized, at least in the beginning. *Certain head motions end up in an approximately 30 second vigorous attack of spinning in the plane of the motion.* As time passes, the paroxysms fade in their intensity but still represent a physical restriction in the life of the patient.

Figure 7.1 shows what goes on in the patient's inner ear.

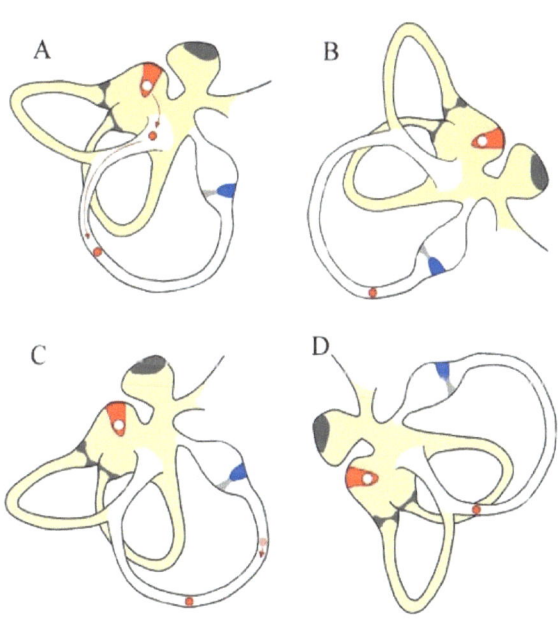

*Figure 7.1. **A**: a small portion of the otoconial membrane (the red dot) loosens and drops (due to gravity) into the inferior canal. **B**: the patient rises from bed and the lump slides down the canal to the lowermost part. **C** and **D**. The lump slides backwards and forwards with head movements. When the lump moves in the canal, it works as a piston more forceful than a normal stimulus which is caused by the inertia of the fluid. The patient experiences a much more than normal rotation, a vertigo fit. Like a backwards or forwards somersault.*

Very often, the patients tell that when trying to get out of the bed in the morning, they feel like they are being thrown around in the bedroom and forced back into bed. At some point the patients must get on their feet. They often try several different strategies and ultimately realize that if their motions are very slow and they take their time to recover from small spinning fits during the rising process, they are able to get on their feet. Walking is not easy because head motions must be avoided. Tooth brushing is difficult and can only be performed with the head still, which is not easy. What do most patients think? *"I have had a cerebral stroke, but I'm awake an able to move with caution. I have no other symptoms, no paralyses; my speech and hearing is preserved, so I will go and see my doctor.*

Often the GP knows about the condition, asks only a few questions, focuses shortly on other symptoms and then performs a provocative test, laying the patient down on one side and then on the other side, head turned 45° to the right, when laid down on the left side, and opposite when laid down on the right side. One of the procedures provokes a half minute long fit of violent vertigo. Then the patient is informed that the disease is absolutely benign, known as *benign positioning vertigo* – and that is curable as soon as the patient is ready to experience a new fit of spinning.

The first maneuver is the diagnostic test called the *Dix-Hallpike maneuver*, see fig. 7.2. Nystagmus will always be part of the picture, at least during the first weeks or months. Nystagmus will appear in the plane of the head movement and involve a rotation of the eye ball and vertical movements as well.

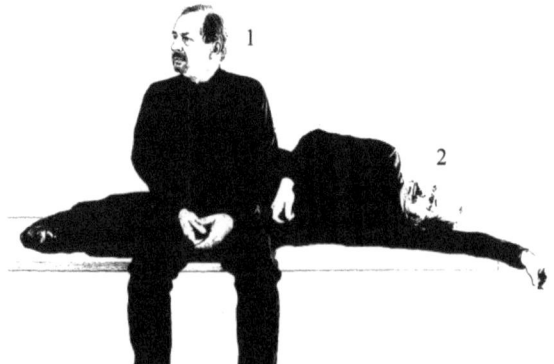

Figure 7.2. The Dix-Hallpike test, modified so that the patient during the maneuver faces the examiner. The **left** *inferior canal is tested. There is vertical/torsional nystagmus accompanying the patient's vertigo.*

The Dix-Hallpike test is testing if there is a freely moving lump of otoconia originating from a fracture in the otolith membrane of the utricle (see fig. 7.1) The next procedure, the GP will perform is the therapeutic procedure which could be an *Epley's maneuver*[3].

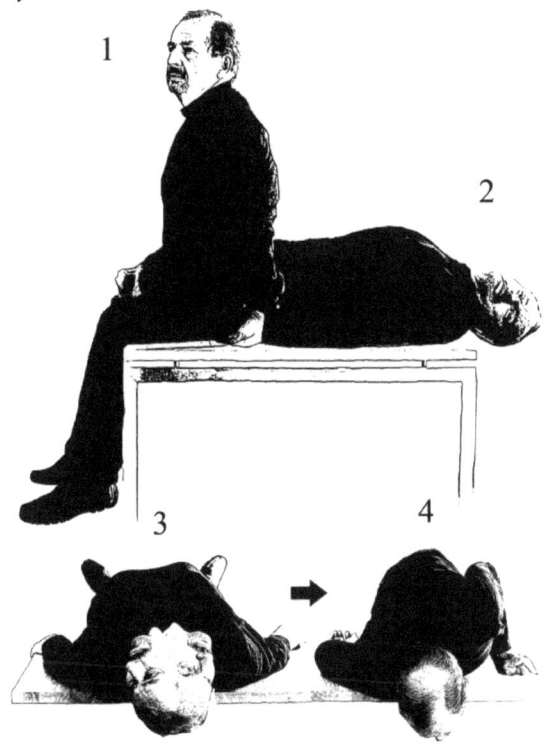

*Figure 7.3. Epley's maneuver, treating BPPV in the **left** inferior semicircular canal. **1**, Turn the head to the left. **2**. Without changing the head orientation lay the patient down on the back. **3→4**. After the disappearance of the vertigo turn the patient (head and body) around until he/she lies with the nose down and maintain the position for 1-2 minutes. When rising again, keep the chin down during the motion.*

At the same time as Epley described his maneuver, a French physiotherapist, *Alain Semont*, published the method named for him.

---

[3] In the late 1980's *John Epley* MD, who is an ear specialist in Portland, Oregon, realized that if a lump of otoconia can get so far because of gravitation, it must be possible to get it back in the utricle using the same physical force.

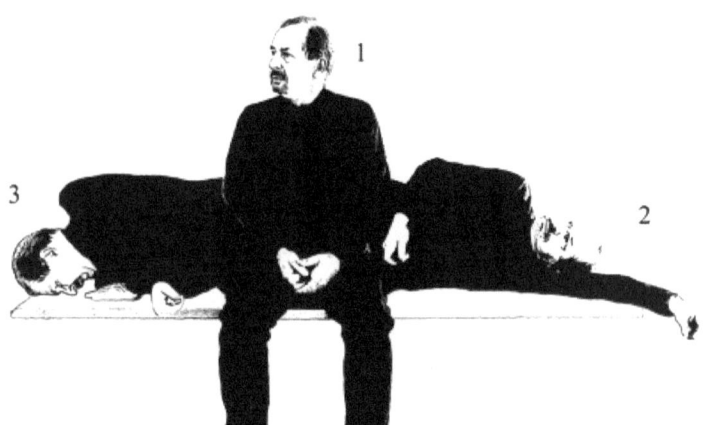

*Figure 7.4. Semont's maneuver for the **left** inferior canal. 1: Patient is sitting, head turned left. 2. Lies down on the left side, still with the head turning left. 3: Throws himself/herself to the right not turning his head.*

Epley's and Semont's maneuvers are based on two different principles. If compared with a person who wants to pass a ball to another person, Epley takes the ball in his hand, walks to the other person and hands the ball to him. It is sure and safe. Semont throws the ball in order to make the other person catch it. Success or failure, you cannot be sure. Semont's maneuver can be performed by the patient himself as many times as it takes to succeed, while Epley's maneuver must be conducted by a helping person in order to be able to pass the point where the patient experiences a maximum of vertigo. During the Epley maneuver, the patient, because of the vertigo fit, as a reflex stops the movement when performing the first part unless a helper's hands guide the head to the hanging position. There will still be a violent vertigo, but the patient relaxes and it is usually possible to complete the maneuver. If the patient has the Epley maneuver twice, there is a more than a 90% chance of success.

Opinions vary about which method to prefer. Regardless of the technique, there is in all cases a great chance to cure the patient.

What happens if the patient has no treatment? There is some evidence suggesting that approximately one third of the BPPV patients heal spontaneously within the first week or two. If the condition does not heal spontaneously, there is a risk of months, even years of suffering. The spontaneous course of the symptoms usually is not a continuation of the violent vertigo fits experienced the first day or weeks of the ailment. The brain slowly learns that those violent somersaults are not real motions. Common

44

sense says "no", the other sensory organs, the superior canal in the opposite ear, the otolith organs, the proprioceptive system, and vision all also deny the story told by the single inferior canal. The vertigo fades somehow and the accompanying nystagmus in many patients disappears. Typically, the patients still feel uneasy during locomotion, often accompanied by some nausea. So the patient does not feel well.

Inferior canal BPPV is the type of BPPV seen most frequently. Looking at fig. 7.1 A, representing a patient lying on the right side, it is evident that the lump of otoconia just as well could have dumped to the horizontal canal. If this happens, there are three possible outcomes:

1. The lump returns to the utricle if the patient spontaneously rolls to the other side during sleep. No vertigo problems.
2. The lump stays in the canal, see fig.7.5. When the patient rolls a little to one side or the other there will some disturbing amplification in the patient's experience of rolling over and back, but this does not challenge the sense of what is up and down, and the patient subconsciously will feel safe lying still in the bed. When getting up, the patient will experience a carousel like, often violent vertigo when moving the head from side to side. By reflex, the patient contracts the muscles and keeps the head as still as possible, only making small movements from side to side. This soon turns into a tender, painful neck. See fig. 7.5 below.

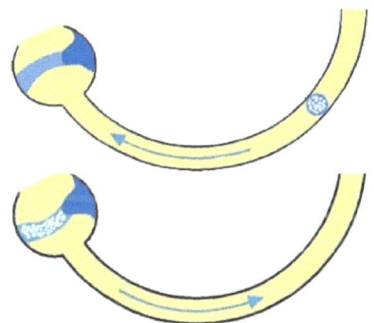

Figure 7.5. Free floating lump of otoconia above (canalolithiasis) and otoconia sticking or absorbed to the cupula (cupulolithiasis) below.

3. The lump stays in the horizontal canal adherent to the cupula of the ampular organ (see fig. 7.5). Normally the cupula is indifferent gravity-wise and it floats in the endolymph, influenced only by the inertia of the endolymph. Now, because the otoconia adds mass to the cupula, the *position* of the cupula will determine the signaling of the organ. The

45

cupula has been transformed into a kind of otolith organ, but still hyper-reacting to rotatory motions. The patient now experiences rotational vertigo when lying on both sides, worst on the opposite side. There will be a nystagmus in the opposite direction of that provoked by a free floating otoconia lump. Nystagmus will be in the direction to the ceiling – a free floating lump will cause a nystagmus to the floor. The two different mechanisms are named differently, when the lump is free floating, it is called *canalolithiasis*, when the otoconia stick to the cupula, it is *cupulolithiasis*. See fig. 7.5 above.

Why this difference between the inferior and horizontal canal BPPV? Gravitational pull is probably to blame. In the inferior canal case the lump stays in the lowermost part of the canal and never comes close to the cupula (compare fig. 7.1). This happens very easily in the case of the horizontal canal. When in touch with the cupula, the otoconia seem to stick to or absorb to the cupula gelatin, which is analogous to the gelatin in the otolith organs.

Canalo- or cupulolithiasis are easily diagnosed by a *supine-roll-test*, see fig. 7.6.

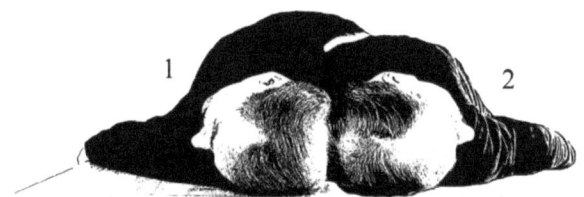

*Figure 7.6. The **supine-roll-test**, testing the **right** horizontal canal, a fast rotation from 1 → 2. If there is a free floating otoconia lump in the canal, the patient will experience a rotational vertigo in the same direction as the movement, if the otoconia stick to the cupula, cupulolithiasis, the direction is opposite. The nystagmus follows the direction of the sensation. Because the stimulus in the cupulolithiasis is not transient as in the canalolithiasis, **both nystagmus and vertigo sensation lasts longer in cupulolithiasis**.*

If a patient suffers from BPPV of the horizontal canal, treatment is easy. If the lump is free floating, it can be forced back into the utricle by letting the patient perform a slow, stepwise 360° rotation direction from the sick side to the opposite side, known as a **barbecue rotation** (a chef would call it a *rôtisserie* rotation). If signs and symptoms point to a cupulolithiasis, the patient has to shake the head violently from side to side for a while to loosen the otoconia,

46

followed by another supine-roll-test to see if the otoconia have loosened from the cupula and turned the disease into a canalolithiasis case – and then a barbecue rotation is performed. It might take a few attempts to reach the canalothiasis condition. The patients should be able to the repeat treatment maneuvers by themselves at home, if taught the methods by the therapist.

It is rare that the superior canal suffers from BPPV. But in the few cases, an inferior canal BPPV is converted to a superior canal BPPV. It may happen during an Epley or Semont maneuver. If lucky, the lump will immediately return to the utricle from the posterior leg of the canal (compare fig 7.1B). If the lump reaches the anterior part of the canal, it will dump into the ampulla and probably stick to or mix up with the cupula. All cases of BPPV in the superior canal are cupulolithiasis cases. They are diagnosed by the Dix-Hallpike test. In the supine position, there will be an upward/torsional nystagmus in contrast to the downward/torsional nystagmus seen in inferior canal BBPV. Since it always is a cupulolithiasis, treatment must start with a loosening procedure, having the patient nodding violently a number of times – and then, when there is a free floating lump of otoconia, a throwing procedure should be performed. The Argentine specialist, Darío Yacovino, has designed the method seen in fig. 7.7 below.

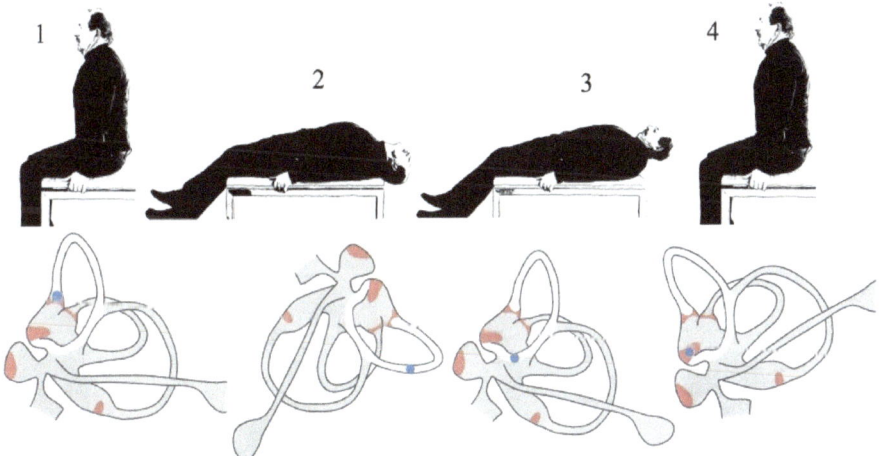

Figure 7.7. Yacovinos maneuver. After having performed the nodding exercise sitting (1), the patient lies down (2), head hanging, and rises quickly into an upright position (3 → 4), adding inertia to the lump that drops down the posterior leg into the utricle. This can be performed a number of times before a successful endpoint. This can be performed by the patient later on, if less successful.

The effort to diagnose and subsequently treat BPPV in patients who describe a sudden, unexpected vertigo is always worthwhile and rewarding. This is the good side of the coin. The reverse side is that the BPPV will reappear in many patients.

Usually, the next time the patient experiences BPPV, he/she will not be as frustrated as the first time, and will know that it is not a cerebral disaster; and they know by experience that the disorder is curable. The risk of having a new BPPV within the first year is high, close to 50%. In cases of recurrence of BPPV, and even at its first appearance, the question of "why" may arise. Something must have gone wrong in the gelatin of the utricle since it has been the victim of a fracture.

In some few cases, it happens as a consequence of a head trauma. A head traumatized patient complaining of dizziness is very often told that the dizziness is a part of the symptoms expected due to a concussion – and that it will disappear over time. But if the condition allows for it, it might ease the patient's suffering if a BPPV is diagnosed and treated already in the emergency room. For reasons unknown, posttraumatic BPPV will have a higher than normal recurrence rate.

It is logical to conclude that something has gone wrong in one inner ear that has not happened in the other ear, since the condition is almost always unilateral/one canal. One explanation for BPPV being unilateral is that it tends to appear on the side on which the patient has the habit of sleeping. For simple anatomical reasons, nothing can dump from the utricle into a canal in the uppermost ear during sleep. But it does not always come in the morning after sleep. Some patients experience the first fit when they are awake during the daytime. The passage from the utricle to a canal could happen because of centrifugal forces during head motions. Centrifugal forces are equal on the left and right side even on a very forceful head rotation. So it still points to the gelatin in just one of the utricles.

Nothing in this world comes from nothing, but in most cases of BPPV it is unclear why a certain person, at a specific time, runs into this problem. There is clearly a higher incidence of BPPV in patients suffering from inner ear diseases, like menière patients, see 7.5 and in patients suffering from migraine, see 7.6.

7.5 Menière's disease

Prosper Menière (1799-1862) was a French ear specialist who worked at the Parisean Institute of Deaf-Mutes. In January 1861, he published a paper in the Gazette Médicale de Paris claiming that a patient suffering from *both hearing problems and dizziness suffered from a disorder of the inner ear*. That was

48

concluded based on his own clinical experience and with reference to observations by his fellow Frenchman, the pioneer physiologist *Pierre Flourens (1794-1867)*. In 1842 Flourens had claimed that the anatomically complex part of the inner ear known as the labyrinth, served balance and orientation. In 1861, Menière read his paper about the significance of the inner ear to the Imperial Academy of Medicine in Paris. His theses were discussed in the academy, of which Menière was *not* a member. Menière's assertion caused fierce opposition from members of the distinguished academy, among them some leading, world-famous neurologists, who told Menière that it was a well-established fact that all kinds of dizziness were caused by accumulation of blood in the brain. A debate continued for the next year and ceased only because Menière died from a pneumonia in January the next year, 1862. Second thoughts are often the consequence of unexpected deaths, even of an opponent. Frontiers softened so much that Menière's opponents declared that Menière possibly was right.

During the academic fight, Menière described a group of patients who complained of having in common three symptoms:

1. Intermittent attacks of vertigo
2. Hearing losses of increasing severity, and
3. Noises in the ear of a variable nature.

A few years later, in 1867, the condition was named *Menière's disease* in honor of his pioneering work.

Due to a common complaint among Menière patients, i.e., fullness of the ear, some considered Menière's disease as a kind of *glaucoma of the inner ear* (glaucoma is a condition of the eye, characterized by an increased pressure in the eye ball and by a progressive loss of vision). In 1938, independent of each other, *Hallpike and Cairns of London* and *Yamakawa of Osaka, Japan* described that there was a severe distension of the membranes of the inner ears of patients suffering from Menière's disease probably due to pressure regulation problems.

Over time there have been varying definitions of the disease, all with clear reference to Menière's observations. Before mentioning the latest definition. I want to state that such definitions are not made for daily clinical purposes, but made in order to present uniform patient samples in scientific publications to make conclusions drawn as valid as possible. Some of these definitions are not very operational in a daily clinical context, and if the aim is to make early diagnosis in order to start relevant treatment as early as possible with the purpose of reducing the overall burden of the disease for the patient, the definitions may be counterproductive by delaying the time of diagnosis.

The following Menière definition is currently accepted and acceptable:

49

A. Two or more spontaneous episodes of vertigo lasting 20 minutes to 12 hours.
B. Audiometrically documented low to medium frequency sensorineural hearing loss in the affected ear on at least one occasion before, during, or after one of the episodes of vertigo.
C. Fluctuating aural symptoms (hearing, tinnitus or fullness in the affected ear.
D. Other causes excluded.

Considering these symptoms, most of the criteria (with the hearing test (audiometry) as an exception) depend alone on the story told by the patient. There are no criteria concerning the vestibular function, partly because there is no accepted standard for vestibular testing, but also because all vestibular parameters, like hearing, vary especially in the first stage of the disease.

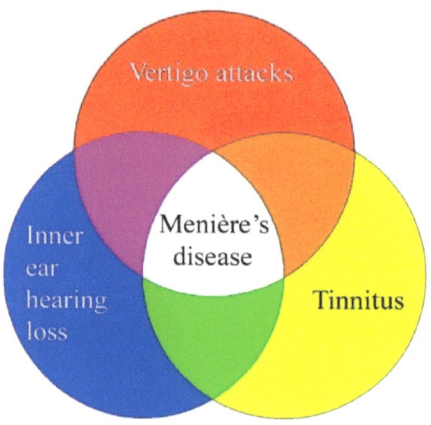

Figure 7.8. The key symptoms of Menière's disease. Very often, the patients also complain of fullness of the ear, indicating a pressure event in the inner ear. All symptoms are of a fluctuating nature. As time passes and if the disease remains active, permanent losses of vestibular function and hearing will appear. The hearing loss is characterized by a simultaneous hypersensitivity to loud sounds and by sound distortion.

Nobody knows what provokes the disease. *We know that migraine patients have a substantially higher risk of having the disease.* We know that some of the patients (approximately 10%) have relatives suffering from the disease. The familial type of Menière's disease is clinically indistinguishable from the much more usual, non-familial cases. Some believe in an autoimmune mechanism (at least for some Menière patients), others do not. In some patients, a hydrops of the inner ear has developed due to some kind of head trauma or inner ear infections, resulting in what is called a *secondary hydrops*. That is all, but the last word about the genetics has yet to be said.

50

Menière's disease is a relatively rare disease. There have been very different estimates varying by time and geography. One of the newest estimates tells that in the US there is 190 Menière patients per 100,000 inhabitants (which should be considered a relatively high estimate), with a rate of women to men of 1.89:1. The onset of the disease typically is in the fifth or sixth decades of life.

There is only one valid statement concerning the individual development of the disease: *it is 100% unpredictable*. Doctors seeing Menière patients realize that the disease is a very heavy burden with respect to quality of life and social opportunities, like maintaining a job. But only the worst stories are reported to doctors. There are probably a large number of patients for whom the disease spontaneously comes to an end after a few attacks without the knowledge or diagnosis by the patient's doctor. There are many cases treated successfully in an early stage. In the other end, there are patients who are forced to give up their occupation and to give up travel and other social activities outside of their homes, including driving a car, to avoid the risk and inconvenience or risks of suffering a vertigo attack under circumstances where they put themselves or others at risk, or where it will be considered embarrassing to suddenly experience what other people might think is a severe alcohol intoxication.

Usually, Menière's disease presents itself as a *unilateral* phenomenon, but there are different opinions about how to define *bilateral* Menière's disease. If sticking to the definition and demanding that there must be evidence that ear number 2 is the origin of vertigo attacks, only a few percent of the patients suffer from a bilateral disease. If looking for other inner ear hearing problems, including tinnitus, to develop over a couple of decades, over 50% will claim that they have developed a problem in the other ear, which at least could be considered the result of similar, but less pronounced inner ear pathology.

Worst of all are the vertigo attacks. These attacks come suddenly, unpredictably, and seemingly unprovoked, often announced by an increased tinnitus and/or fullness of the ear a few minutes before. In almost all cases the patient is forced to lie down, very often for hours. In seconds or minutes after the onset, the patient will start experience nausea and many patients will vomit. There may be an increasing tinnitus in the diseased ear and in many patients a severe transient deafness. Since the patient feels better lying with the diseased ear facing upward, communication with the patient is difficult. The patient feels extremely sick. Spectators are not in doubt – the patient is almost as sick as possible. Vertigo worsens if the patient moves or is moved. Any activity around the patient is unpleasant. Spectators scared of what is happening will typically call for an ambulance to bring the patient to the nearest emergency facility. The staff at the hospital, if uncertain about what is happening, will cause further discomfort for the patient if they conduct a cerebral scan. If it is the patient's first attack, the patient too is unaware of the nature of the disease and unable to tell people that it is an ear disease and not a brain disaster.

The unexperienced patient having the first Menière attack, not knowing if the attack will ever stop, may accept procedures, which the experienced patient knows are unnecessary and very unpleasant. In the case of a cerebral scan, the patient will be forced to move into the scanner and lie still on the back, which is very unpleasant for the patient and if impossible, counterproductive for any scanning procedure. It would be nice if all emergency personnel knew about Menière's disease and were able to recognize a Menière attack when presented with it. The key is the violent vertigo and nystagmus any direction or direction changing, and the unilateral ear and hearing symptoms, and that there are no signs or symptoms of CNS disorder.

In some patients (less than 10%), another type of vertigo attack will develop during their active disease. The attacks are named after a British doctor, *A. Tumarkin*, who in 1936 described the phenomenon. The patient suddenly falls, feeling as if they are pushed or shoved to the ground, or they fall because their surroundings suddenly move or tilt. The attacks are called *Tumarkin's otolithic crises* or *vestibular drop attacks*. There is no loss of consciousness. The attacks come suddenly out of nowhere and the fall may result in unpleasant lesions, depending on where and how they happen. The episodes are extremely stressful. They are probably caused by a sudden loss of function of an otolith organ leading to a loss of control over the muscles counteracting gravity.

For a lot of Menière patients, there is one phenomenon independently of the type and strength of the attacks, that is worse than the attacks themselves - not knowing when they can expect the next attack. Attacks rarely come regularly.

Whatever provokes an attack is unknown. Inner ear microscopy of preparations from patients who have passed away for any other reason show that it is very often obvious that there have been ruptures of the inner ear membranes. Because of that, it seems plausible that a membrane rupture could provoke an attack. A blending of peri- and endolymph will discharge the inner ear of the electric potential across the membrane, and we know that a sudden loss of vestibular function will result in a severe vertigo attack, see fig. 7.9, and compare fig. 3.1.

52

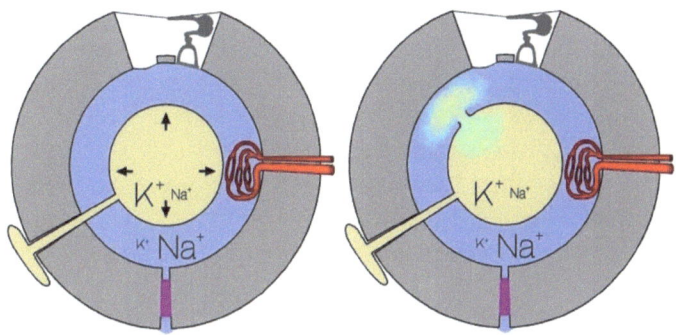

Figure 7.9. The rupture theory. A rupture of the membrane will result in a blending of peri- and endolymph resulting in a discharging of the electric potential across the membrane. Compare with fig. 3.1.

If a permanent loss of vestibular function occurs with time, and it does in most long lasting cases, it will result in a permanent imbalance and unsteadiness.

Characteristically, the hearing fluctuates. For some patients it will continue to do so for the entire time there is Menière activity in the ear. The hearing may be fluctuant independent of the vertigo attacks. This is very tiresome for the patient, not knowing how their hearing will perform in a matter of hours from now. The hearing may be normal between the first attacks, but with time it usually worsens. It will be dominated by deteriorations, distortion and sound hypersensitivity. A phenomenon called *recruitment of loudness* is more or less present in all ears suffering from an inner ear hearing loss. It is best described by grandpa's statement: "don't shout, I'm not deaf". Yes, he's deaf the old guy, but he suffers from a hypersensitivity to loud sounds. So if you want to pass a message to the old man, you must use a clear, medium volume voice and tell the other family members to keep their communication at quieter level; grandpa's ears have problems discriminating words in a noisy environment. This is also the case for a Menière patient.

With progression of the hearing loss, it might end up with a non-serviceable hearing state, meaning that no hearing aid will help the patient. Fitting a hearing aid is difficult or impossible if the hearing fluctuates. Since most patient have a normal or at least significantly better hearing on the other ear, they become very critical hearing aid users (they can compare sound quality of the two ears) and often prefer to live without a hearing aid. Further, it is difficult for a hearing aid to compensate for the distortion part of the hearing problem.

As in other inner ear diseases, tinnitus tends to increase with increased hearing loss. Tinnitus in Menière's disease also has its own agenda. Often it is loudest during the attacks, but definitely not as troublesome as the usually extremely violent vertigo. A lot of Menière patients have a very forgiving relationship with their tinnitus; there are more severe symptoms to care about. Approximately 80% of the patients consider the *fullness* sensation an important symptom. For some Menière patients, it is not a predominant symptom. For others, it is a great embarrassment. If it is bad, it is felt like a deep pain in the ear.

There are a large number of *treatment options*. This indicates that there is no single treatment with a universal healing effect. Traditionally, treatment has focused on low salt/diuretic regimes, originating from a theory that the pressure load on the inner ear will be eased that way. Since the mid-1970th, betahistine, a specific Menière drug, has been widely used, especially in Europe. This is a histamine-like drug dispensed in tablet form. It was developed because intravenous histamine-therapy had gained popularity and intravenous treatment is costly and unpleasant. In spite of its popularity, it has been impossible, to finally prove its efficacy in larger state-of-the-art clinical trials.

A minimally invasive treatment such as inserting a *ventilation tube* into the ear drum may help some patients. It seems to be that some Menière patients have a larger than normal spontaneous negative pressure variation in their *middle* ears. These variations seem to have an impact on the *inner ear* pressure regulation. If small positive pressure impulses are applied to the Menière ear by means of a device called a Meniett®, some patients feel comfort and report that their disease is under control.

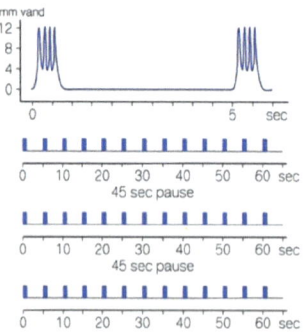

Figure 7.10. The pressure waves produced by the Meniett® device.

Other and more dramatic irreversible surgical and medical methods may be used if the above mentioned treatment options are insufficient in controlling

54

the disease, with control of the violent vertigo attacks as the main target of all treatments.

For years, *labyrinthectomy*, the surgical destruction of the inner ear, has ultimately been used if no other treatment seemed sufficient. The price to be paid for the patient is that the he/she must learn to live without any hearing at all in the diseased ear and must try to compensate for the loss of vestibular function in that ear. Very often, there is so much remaining function before surgery, both hearing- and balance-wise, that the patient will suffer from the procedure. Vestibular compensation is always partial, and in some patients so insufficient that patients end up in a wheelchair. The procedure will not improve patients' tinnitus. A specific vestibular effect can be obtained by cutting only the vestibular nerve. It does not change the hearing, and like following a labyrinthectomy, there is no risk for more vertigo attacks.

Other treatment options have been searched for to reduce the burden of loss of sensory function. One of them is a kind of "chemical warfare" solution. A small volume of a gentamicin (see 7.3.2) is inserted through the ear drum into the middle ear, to be absorbed to the inner ear through the two windows. This is meant to paralyze the vestibular organs, the semicircular canals and the otolith organs. If handled carefully, hearing will be preserved in most patients, and in a few patients even some of the vestibular function, so the patient usually will be better off compared to destructive surgery. Some doctors aim at a vestibular paralysis, others wait and see what happens after one or two injection and stays ready to supply more gentamicin if the treatment seems insufficient.

Since this treatment option has become popular, other drugs than gentamicin have been tried. There is evidence that some Menière patients benefit from steroid (cortisone) treatment. It is difficult to accept the side effect of a long term, high dosage cortisone therapy. This can be avoided by installing steroids into the middle ear, as done with gentamicin, usually performed repeatedly with a few days or weeks interval. The final word has yet to be said about this treatment.

One very important treatment is to establish a confidential, sufficiently long lasting patient-doctor relationship between the Menière patient and the doctor taking care of the patient. Many Menière patients have stated that the simple fear of having an attack can become a potential provocation of the next attack. So no wonder it is difficult to prove for certain that a treatment any kind is more efficient than a placebo treatment – in both cases the patient feels good being taking care of. The cyclic behavior of the disease, the patient seeking help when the disease is causing most trouble, is another confounder.

In Menière's disease, the fear of the next attack should be considered a relevant treatment criteria.

7.6 Vestibular migraine

For centuries, it has been known that there is a link between dizziness and migraine. In his 1861-paper, Prosper Menière mentioned that symptoms described as those seen in what later became known as Menière's disease, often are seen in migraine patients. Only recently (in 2012), a specific name and diagnostic criteria were decided for in a joint action of the *Bárány Society* (the leading international society of vestibular research) and the *International Headache Society* and then registered in the latter society's *International Classification of Headache Disorders (ICHD)*. The disease was named *vestibular migraine* and a subgroup of vestibular migraine, *probable vestibular migraine* was also defined by the following criteria:

1. Vestibular migraine:
A. At least 5 episodes with vestibular symptoms of moderate or severe intensity, lasting 5 minutes to 72 hours
B. Current or previous history of migraine with or without aura, according to the International Classification of Headache Disorders (ICHD).
C. One or more migraine features with at least 50% of the vestibular episodes:
  – headache with at least two of the following characteristics: one sided, pulsating quality, moderate or severe pain intensity, aggravation by routine physical activity
  – photophobia or phonophobia
  – visual aura
D. Not better accounted for by another vestibular or ICHD diagnosis.

2. Probable vestibular migraine:
A. At least 5 episodes with vestibular symptoms of moderate or severe intensity, lasting 5 minutes to 72 hours
B. Only one of criteria B and C for vestibular migraine fulfilled (migraine history or migraine features during the episode)
C. Not better accounted for by another vestibular or ICHD diagnosis

As in the case of Menière's disease, criteria are not made for daily clinical purposes, but in order to have uniform patient samples in different scientific publications to make conclusions drawn as valid as possible.

It is not a violation of any law to fit a patient, not fulfilling all the accepted criteria, into the diagnosis. It is not uncommon to do so for patients never

56

having had a migraine headache if the patient has a clear family history of migraine.

Vestibular migraine is considered one of *the most common causes of episodic vertigo*. All experts agree that the condition is very much underdiagnosed. It is estimated that 1% of the population suffers from vestibular migraine, which make the disease significantly more common than Menière's disease. There are more women than men suffering from vestibular migraine, up to five times as many, some estimates say.

In *children*, migraine-related syndromes are also the most common cause of vertigo and dizziness. If vertigo or dizziness is the only symptom, the condition is named *benign paroxysmal vertigo in childhood*. It usually begins before school age and disappears by itself a few years later. It may be accompanied by headaches. Attacks are accompanied by nystagmus and may be brief, leaving the patient with a headache.

In adults very short attacks of vestibular migraine are common. The five minutes lower limit of the duration of attacks from the definition paper seems too long for some patients. The duration of attacks may be described by patients as a constant feeling of unsteadiness with vertiginous exacerbations provoked by visually moving objects or flicker, e.g. as experienced when working at a computer station. Some other patients describe vertigo attacks of a severity that make them resemble those in Menière's disease but most patients describe attacks of a severity much less, attacks only calling for a short break in their activities. Attacks may be accompanied by sound hypersensitivity and hypersensitivity to light and smells. *Many patients feel that unsteadiness or unbalance is their worst daily problem.* Some patients feel that they are able to gain full control over their dizziness when exercising (e.g., running) and that the dizziness returns immediately afterward, at even higher levels than before the exercise.

There is no doubt that there is a broad transition zone between vestibular migraine and Menière's disease. In some cases, the migraine vertigo mimics Menière's disease so much that a diagnosis like *"Menière's light"* is tempting. Differences between Menière's disease and vestibular migraine often are:

1. Hearing loss and ear symptoms are well defined and unilateral in Menière's.
2. If the migraine patient complains of hearing symptoms, they often are bilateral; there may be a hypersensitivity and distortion of sounds, more than a deafness. This might persist between attacks, as in Menière's.

3. Very often the migraine patient suffers from tinnitus, often equally in both ears, in contrast to the one-ear tinnitus typically for the Menière patient.
4. As mentioned above the severity of vertigo attacks is much higher in Menière patients.
5. Aural pressure or fullness is present in many vestibular migraine patients, often in both ears simultaneously or alternating left and right.

We know that migraine attacks may change into a clear cut Menière's disease in some patients. This happens in a few postmenopausal women having suffered from migraine – and it may change back into headaches, if the patient is treated with estrogens.

Objective vestibular findings in vestibular migraine are variable, with most prominent variability in otolith organ function (VEMP tests) – just like in the early stage of Menière's disease. Conventional audiometry in migraine usually is normal in contrast to the low to middle frequency hearing loss typically found in most Menière patients. The character of the vestibular complaints also points more at an otolith dysfunction than at the semicircular canal as *agent provocateur*. Patients often suffer more from a balance problem than from a spinning feeling.

Evidence of familiarities between the two conditions is overwhelming. So why not conclude that a condition that involves both vestibular and auditory functions is an inner ear problem and not a brain problem? Prosper Menière, at least, would agree from his resting place in the Montparnas Cemetery in Paris. Provoking mechanisms are present, but often unknown in both conditions, and they might indeed originate from the brain.

External dietary provoking factors are found in some patients, but only if one is looking for them. Often they are easy to exclude from the patient's diet and this is may be a successful countermeasure. In women, obvious patterns of symptoms may appear in time with a hormonal "event", e.g. with menstruation, when starting oral contraception, when ending oral contraception, with insertion of a hormonal IUD, or the removal of one. In such cases, it is logical to try to return to the pre-symptom hormonal state if possible. If it is a postmenopausal phenomenon, why not consider a hormonal substitution, as mentioned above.

If none of these dietary or hormonal interventions are successful, medical treatment should be considered as the next measure. Attack therapy may be tried using the same drugs as used in migraine headaches, e.g., the *triptans*. In some patients these work, but the number of patient is definitely less than those who claim that they are useless.

The world of *prophylactic drug intervention* is as complex as it is in migraine headaches. All the medication options are loaded with adverse effects, very often being dizziness of a different kinds, as with *β-blockers* – they lower the blood pressure, which may cause dizziness of the fainting type, as one of several not very pleasant adverse effects. Some *antiepileptics*, e.g., vaproic acid and topiramate, are also loaded with side effects, among them also dizziness. A *calcium-blocker*, flunarizine, is used by some. Some doctors recommend *tricyclic antidepressants*, e.g., amitriptryline and nortriptyline, also drugs with a number of adverse effects. Tricyclic antidepressants are used in doses far below those used as antidepressant therapy, they might be helpful in some patients (in low doses, it is not an antidepressant therapy). A relatively old *antihistamine/anti-motion sickness drug, cinnarizine*, has been in trial and might show up as a solution in some patients. In all cases, it may take some time to find out for a certain patient which drug in which dose is the treatment of choice. In most cases drug trials claiming effects are not of the scientifically valuable type, namely randomized, and double-blinded, so conclusions drawn from such trials are not very safe.

We need to have much more focus on the treatment aspects of vestibular migraine. The relatively new definition criteria will probably help future drug trials to become more conclusive.

Vestibular rehabilitation is important in all cases of dizziness. It eases the cerebral interpretation of conditions of peripheral and central dysfunction and trains and maintains the muscular-sensory interaction so important for balance function.

A much broader understanding of the biological mechanisms behind the disorder could ease the search for treatment options. In that sense vestibular migraine is not different from other disorders.

7.7 Other conditions causing dizziness and vertigo due to inner ear dysfunction.

7.7.1 The tensor tympani syndrome (controversial topic)

Two minor muscles in the middle ear, the *stapedius muscle* and the *tensor tympani muscle*, when working together reduce harmful noise effects on the inner ear by increasing the resistance in the middle ear sound transmission system. The stapedius muscle contraction produces a pull backwards of the stapes and the tensor muscle pulls forward in the hammer and tighten ups the ear drum, see the fig. 7.11. Part of the tensor tympani muscle is contained in the bony canal of the auditory tube (Eustachian tube).

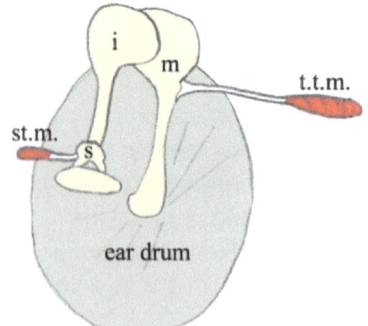

Figure 7.11. The middle ear muscles and the inside of the ear drum seen from the tympanic cavity inwards out. **st.m.** *is the stapedial muscle,* **t.t.m.** *the tensor tympani muscle.* **s**, **i**. *and* **m**. *are the middle ear bones, the auditory ossicles: the stapes, the incus and the malleus.*

The stapedial muscle is activated by loud sounds (> 85 dB). When contracted, it will result in an immediate reflex contraction of the tensor muscle, reacting to almost any disturbance.

The *tensor tympani syndrome* will appear if the tensor tympani muscle is allowed to work by itself, producing a pull on and distortion of the middle ear bones, resulting in a movement of the stapes not counteracted by the stapedial muscle. The stapes movement will cause a pressure wave in the inner ear, experienced as a click-sound. An independent activation of the tensor tympani muscle is made possible because it may contract in time with activities in the mastication muscles.

The main symptoms of the syndrome are hypersensitivity to sound, tinnitus, unsteadiness, and dizziness.

People who suffer from bruxism (the habit of grinding the teeth while asleep) will produce pressure waves to the inner with a potential harmful effect, causing typical inner ear symptoms. The first to describe the problem was a Swedish audiologist, *Ingvar Klockhoff MD of Uppsala*, in the 1960's. So the syndrome is also called the *Klockhoff syndrome*. There are theories that link the syndrome with Menière's disease, postulating that the tensor tympani contractions might stress the inner ear and cause the development of an endolymphatic hydrops.

The simplest treatment option, if bruxism is causing troubles, is to sleep with a bite guard thus stopping the grinding of the teeth. In all cases, a dentist subspecialized in bite function disorders should be involved.

7.7.2 Dehiscense of the superior canal

The *Tullio phenomenon*, a symptom named after the Italian physiologist Pietro Tullio, (1881-1941) has been known for many years. The symptoms are short vertigo fits provoked by sounds. Prior to 1998, not much was known about the

60

phenomenon except for the fact that when surgically exploring the middle ear of patients suffering from Tullio's phenomenon a dangling loose stapes could be seen. The treatment recommendation then was to try mechanically to stabilize the stapes. Some patients benefitted a little from the surgery for at least for a period of time.

In 1998, an American ear specialist, Professor *Lloyd Minor MD*, found an explanation for the phenomenon, a soft tissue separation of the membranes of the brain and the superior semicircular canal, established because of an absence of normal bone above the canal, see fig. 7.12 below. "Dehiscense" means a cleft. Seen from above, the upper surface of the petrous part of the temporal bone at the site of the canal looks like a cleft, missing the dome-like bony appearance of the site of the summit of the canal.

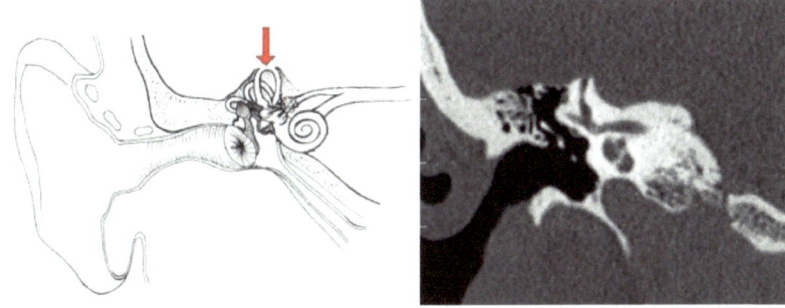

Figure 7.12. A dehiscence of the right superior canal, sketched left and as seen by a CAT-scan right.

The mechanism of the vertigo is that, instead of a one-way direction of the traveling wave caused by the sound via stapes from the oval to the round window, there is another escape of the sound energy through the superior semicircular canal to the new window at the summit of the canal. This is called a "third window effect" to illustrate that the sound energy is converted into a vestibular canal stimulus. Except for the vertigo claims, the patients very often feel that their ear has become very sound sensitive, some are even able to hear their *eyes* move! Sounds transmitted by the bones of the skull seem amplified.

Probably the dangling stapes appears because of vibrations caused by pulsations and other pressure phenomena around the brain induce a sloshing behavior of the perilymph loosening the otherwise tight joint of the stapes.

Most dehiscence patients can be cured by a surgical procedure sealing the superior canal.

7.7.3 Perilymphatic fistula (another controversial topic)

A fistula means an abnormal passage between two otherwise separated hollow anatomical structures. A perilymphatic fistula is a leak allowing perilymph to escape from the perilymphatic space into the middle ear. The condition exists under four different conditions referred to with an increasing degree of controversy among ear surgeons:

1. In a kind of a relatively rare chronic middle ear disease known as cholesteatoma, the collection of debris in the cavity behind the middle ear may "eat" away the bone covering the horizontal semicircular canal, this results in a fistula, in worst and rare cases ending up as inner ear infection (labyrinthitis, see 7.7.4).

2. Fistulae appearing as a consequence of a sudden pressure shift in the middle ear. In diving medicine this is a well-known but rare traumatic condition. In worst case divers present themselves with a sudden maximal hearing loss and maximal vertigo following a problematic forced middle ear pressure clearance during the initial descent of a dive (always within the first ten meters = 33'). It has also been described in air crew, appearing during the descent of the aircraft. Very often, divers or flight crew suffering from a common cold, have felt an urge to dive or fly even though it seemed risky.

   This type of fistula patients must have emergency surgery if symptoms are severe, in order to rescue their hearing and vestibular function. Their round window membranes and the stapes footplate must be sealed to gain control over hearing and balance.

3. Fistula as a complication to middle ear surgery, especially surgery involving pathology of the stapes.

4. The most controversial: perilymphatic fistulae caused by head traumas. The theory of this type of fistulae is that, if exposed to a severe direct head trauma or a whiplash trauma, the inertia of the brain will cause the brain to collide with the inner surface of the skull. The elastic brain will lose volume by the compression and this will result in a displacement of the cerebrospinal fluid (CSF) surrounding the brain, applying suction to all membranes surrounding the CSF). This includes a negative pressure wave to the canal named *cochlear aqueduct* (see fig. 3.1) resulting in a displacement of the loose connective tissue filter in the canal, that under normal conditions protects the inner ear from pressure variations in the CSF. The connective tissue plug then ends up in the CSF, now allowing pressure changes around the brain to alter the inner ear pressure and putting the round window membrane and the joint around the stapes footplate at

risk of bursting. There are observations that support a third location of fistula, a bursting of the usually very thin bony tissue in the center of the stapes footplate. The loss of a protection against a free floating of CSF from the brain through the aqueduct to the perilymphatic space and from there to the middle ear will result in pressure alterations in the inner ear when straining under physical exercise, lifting heavy burdens, and during toilet visits – according to what the patients claim. Further, the inner ear becomes sensitive to middle ear pressure and to loud sounds (the Tullio phenomenon). The nature of the dizziness compares better with disturbance of otolith function than the semicircular canal function.

If fistula surgery is performed under local anesthesia, even small, innocent manipulations of the middle ear bones will provoke dizziness, which is not what happens in common non-fistula ear surgery.

If it is a precondition for the healing that the connective tissue plug regenerates. Postoperative rest is a necessity. Surgery is not always indicated. Some patients heal as a result of a resting regime, avoiding provoking their dizziness by straining, etc.

7.7.4 Labyrinthitis.
As mentioned above (7.7.3), labyrinthitis may be a complication to a chronic inner ear condition, the cholesteatoma, showing up as a violent dizziness and loss of hearing in an ear already suffering from a middle ear infection. The symptoms are attributed to an inner ear infection seen as a progression of a middle infection, usually chronic of nature and often in a cholesteatoma ear and almost always in an already discharging ear. It is a rare condition demanding a fast intervention, involving antibiotics and acute surgery.

7.8 Fainting
Fainting is both losing consciousness and a feeling that it might happen any moment. Everybody knows what it is to feel a blurring of vision, of brightness, and clearness, calling for immediate action to sit down, head between knees, or to lie down, head down, feet high to reestablish cerebral blood circulation. Dizziness is part of the symptoms, loss of balance, too. Always synchronous with disturbance of consciousness,

As bipedal individuals (head high, feet on the ground) arterial blood to the brain is pumped vertically against gravity. The consequence of the vertical anatomy is that organs above heart level demand for a sufficiently high arterial blood pressure, and organs below must transport venous blood to the heart fighting the gravitational pull. The first problem is solved by a feedback of information of arterial pressure from sensory organs in the arteries of the neck, the *carotid sinuses*. The latter is solved by a large number of valves in our leg veins and a firm, elastic fascia-covering of the muscles of the legs, which together make the legs work much like a heart. When muscles in our lower extremities contract for a moment, venous blood within the fascia-stocking is moved from one level to a higher level in the veins, and the valves of the veins prevent the blood from returning to a lower level. If the venous blood does not return to the heart to be oxidized and recirculated, the heart will remain unemployed and blood circulation is obstructed. A parade soldier forced to maintain the position of attention for a while is forced to cheat a little, shifting the weight from one leg to the other (see fig. 3.6D). If he forgets about it, he will soon be an on his back collapsed, unconscious soldier. Now in a supine position, the blood will circulate horizontally, a much easier task for heart, and the parade soldier will wake up again.

This physiology will work well if all elements work. A number of conditions may hamper the procedure:

1. Heart disorders: e.g., a slow or very high pulse rate, attacks of rhythm disturbances, heart insufficiency.
2. Neurologic conditions: peripheral neuropathies, hypersensitive carotid sinus.
3. Drugs, especially those lowering the blood pressure, either according to the purpose of the medication or as a side effect. Some drugs other than anti-hypertensives cause as a side effect a low blood pressure or block the nerve mediated heart response to a falling blood pressure.
4. Low blood pressure as a result of exaggerated exercise. It sounds strange, but just as exercise will lower a too high blood pressure and save patients from anti-hypertensive medication, it tends to generally lower the blood pressure in people with a normal or already low pressure. There is one cure for that: combine running exercise with muscle strengthening (also a WHO recommendation) – that is what is demanded for high performance fighter pilots. If the pilot does not do that, his G-tolerance will diminish and he will faint during a high-G maneuver, like a tight turn. After all, fainting for non-pilots is usually about our 1-G tolerance.
5. Habitual low blood pressure. Some people are blessed by nature by a low blood pressure. They faint more easily than others.
6. A low pressure may also be the result of dehydration leading to a reduction of the blood volume.
7. High fever. If a person has not experienced fainting, just try to rush out of bed with a high fever.

8. Unpleasant experiences. Fainting may appear in some people as a result of unpleasant events, seeing blood, sudden pains or other sensations. It is called a *vasovagal reaction* and considered a normal phenomenon.
9. Hyperventilation. Fainting may be a result of hyperventilation or holding the breath, the secret in the past of many upper-class women, if ignored by their husband during parties.

The examination of a patient suffering from fainting problem involves a drug history, screening for heart disorders, neurological examination and blood sampling to exclude neuropathies caused by diabetes, vitamin B_{12} or other metabolic disease.

In the end (or as a part of the examination at any time), a fainting patient can have the predisposition to fainting (orthostatic reactions) directly tested by a tilt table test, recording pulse rate, blood pressure and ECG during a slow 70° tilt on a motorized table. This test may give indications on where to search for an explanation of fainting.

7.9 Dizziness caused by diseases of the central nervous system

The CNS is not only a relay station of the balance reflexes, it also accounts for the learning processes and plasticity of the balance system (see 3.3.4). But first of all, it plays a ghost role when talking about dizziness. Because normal balance in a narrow sense is an unconscious function, there is a clear and very often false sender's message when a dysfunction of the balance system arises. Maybe because of the brain fog associated with fainting appears together with dizziness, most patients will conclude that dizziness and vertigo is cause by brain dysfunction. In less severe cases, patients and witnesses, most often mistakenly, conclude that the dizzy condition could be caused by dehydration, also referring to the fainting phenomenon.

It is often said that arteriosclerosis of the brain is a common cause of dizziness in elderly, forgetting that arteriosclerosis of the brain will also at the same time cause a number of other neurologic symptoms, as impediment of speech, paralysis of the muscles and sensory disturbances. The same accounts for strokes. If balance is the only symptom, it is probably not a brain problem. Most balance reflexes are fast - when fast, the neuronal circuit must be relatively simple. What is complex with the balance is the sensory integration, the learning processes, and the plasticity of the system, and these functions may be harmed, if cerebral circulation is suffering. Then it is not an acute dysfunction, but a progressive process. If a thrombosis or a hemorrhage hits the brainstem in the form of stroke, a sudden death will be the most likely result, because vital functions like respiration, circulation, and consciousness are all under control of centers in the brainstem.

Multiple sclerosis may produce very small and specific lesions in the brainstem or cerebellum giving rise to a loss of specific functions as the control of eye movements, e.g., related to the smooth pursuit reflex or the saccades, easily seen if relevant tests are performed. There is one important exception. A *thrombosis in the cerebellum* may cause a very specific lesion giving rise to dizziness or vertigo only.

Tumors of the brain follow the same rules as dysfunction of circulation – generally dizziness will not be the only symptom. There is still one exception, some rare tumors of the cerebellum.

The only symptom combination guaranteeing an inner ear disorder and excluding brain disease is, according to Prosper Menière, the combination of hearing problems and balance problems.

If a combination of dizziness and other symptoms cause a suspicion of a CNS disorder, the patient needs a neurologist consultation and a cerebral scan.

Another much more frequent condition indicating brain scans is patient's fear of cerebral disease – even in cases where everything points at the inner ear. *The doubt of the patient is a sufficient indication for brain imaging.*

7.10 Dizziness in the elderly population

With increasing age, the frequency of dizziness complaints increases too. There are good reasons for that, but to blame age alone is not fair, even though many people think and say that it is normal.

Explanations are:

1. Naturally, elderly people are not protected against and will suffer from most of the same diseases as the younger population. In some cases, the prevalence might be even higher, as it is the case with BPPV.
2. There are at least three different explanations why the prevalence of some diseases are higher in an elderly population:
   a. When an individual has lived a long life, minor lesions and wear and tear on the body will sum up, proportionally to age.
   b. With increasing age, nature has decided that degeneration of sensory organs appear (named *multiple sensory system failure*) well known in vision and hearing, but also in the vestibular organs. The number of sensory cells in both otolith organs and semicircular canals will decline.
   c. Other organ functions suffer too: heart, kidneys, muscles, joints, etc.
3. Because of the above mentioned phenomena, elderly people very often are uncritically medicated to compensate for diseases or organ dysfunctions. Drugs are metabolized at a slower rate than in younger people and tend to accumulate. This is comparable to overdosing, even if recommended drug doses are used. This phenomenon of drug overdosing is usually well

considered, if the patient is child, where body size (actually body surface) serves as a guideline for calculating how much of a certain drug should be prescribed. It is not that easy in the elderly population. The risk of overdosing both concerns the desired action of the drug (e.g., anti-hypertensive drugs) and undesired side effects.

Further, the elderly population more readily accepts authority and are less inclined to question the opinions of their doctors.

Many elderly people are prescribed a number of different drugs at the same time. Drugs may interact, e.g., competing for protein carriers in the blood. There is relatively detailed knowledge about the risk of interaction of two-drug combinations, but as the number of drugs taken increases, the risk of adverse effects increases exponentially, in time with a decreasing documentation of safety. There is focus on the risk of *polypharmacy*, but still it is unsafely practiced in too many patients, with a higher risk in older rather than younger patients.

Falls appear more frequently with age. The reasons for this has been mentioned earlier. As we age, the sensory systems degrade, the anti-stumbling reflex degrades due to vision problems, slowing of reflexes, there is a reduction in muscle mass and strength, and maybe a reduced alertness to obstacles. *Vestibular rehabilitation and training is the best cure.*

7.11 Dizziness caused by psychogenic problems and psychological symptoms caused by a somatic balance system dysfunction

There are a number of reasons or excuses for attributing dizziness to psychological dysfunction, and sometimes, indeed, it is well-founded. On the other hand, if a medical person is confronted with a patient with dizziness, immediately concluding himself/herself that there must be a psychological base for the symptoms (as a high stress load for example) it is tempting for the doctor to agree and prescribe a reduction of stress factors and/or a tranquillizer. Will the patient be happier then? Maybe, for a while. Will the patient be cured? Hardly. What's the problem with psychogenic dizziness?

1. *Lack of words*, unclear terminology because the complaints relate to a *non-conscious sensory system*. It is not only the lack of words - it is sometimes as profound as a loss of notion. The sensation of dizziness might be as specific as a sensation of being turned around or being onboard a ship – without any notion of being moved. Often it is less specific: no clear motion but a feeling of distance, bewilderedness. In both cases, what the patient feels seems unreal. *For the patient* the question arises: What's

happening? I'm not the same person as before. The world has changed and I have lost orientation. Am I going crazy? *To the spectator*: a person, usually reacting and speaking meaningfully is now saying strange words and seeking shelter. Going crazy? *To the doctor* with less experience in dizziness: two options. Option one: crazy. Option two: I don't understand and I don't know - potentially desperate signal to convey to the patient. *Probably a stress related condition.* And it is stressful.

2. If things are not what they use to be, we use our defense strategies and they are leading to *anxiety*. Anxiety may physically be very real – if I try to stand on my feet or try to move, I may fall and get hurt.

   *Anxiety may have the very **physiological** form as it has for a moment if you are climbing a ladder and step on a loose rung.* You immediately get a lump in the stomach and your hands become clammy. If this happens every time you try to move, anxiety will be there all the time and the diagnosis *panic anxiety* is close because the patient will panic. The tendency to develop this reaction is very typical in otolith dysfunction. Not knowing what is up and down and losing the opportunity of standing and moving safely on the feet is a big existential crisis. There is a diagnostic entity covering that situation: *phobic postural vertigo*. It takes only a few minutes to explain a patient what is really happening. For a doctor to prescribe a tranquillize takes no time at all – but might be classified as a coward's reaction. If the doctor's explanation is inadequate, the help of a psychologist familiar with the specific type of reaction is needed. *By the way, the most common side effect of tranquillizers is dizziness, so it may come out as a self-fulfilling prophecy!*

3. If motion is associated with dizziness, most patients will develop signs and the cascade of *symptoms characteristic of motion sickness*:
   a. Headaches
   b. Drowsiness
   c. ***Depression***
   d. Nausea
   e. Retching
   f. Vomiting

Frustration is almost always present in dizzy patients. Frustrations of becoming sick, frustration of not having a diagnosis or a reasonable explanation, frustrations of having no relevant or efficient treatment, and frustrations that nobody can guarantee that this is not a lifelong problem.

What is stated above does not mean that a psychotic or neurotic patient would not use the word "dizziness" meaningfully in other contexts. It could be a complaint of a drug side effect, but after all, psychogenic conditions do not protect the patients from other (e.g., vestibular) disorders. If the dizziness-word is used in context with a number of other complaints of doubtless psychogenic nature, it should be interpreted otherwise than described above.

Acknowledgements:

My beloved wife Eva (who is also an ear-nose-throat surgeon), has been very helpful and supportive during the writing process, so have other family members too, including my nurse daughter, Majken and my psychiatrist sister-in-law, Ulla. I am extremely grateful for that.

A native American scholar, Joyce Kling PhD, Postdoctoral Fellow at the University of Copenhagen has perused the manuscript and polished my English. I am deeply grateful to her too.

INDEX